State of AA Research & Treatment

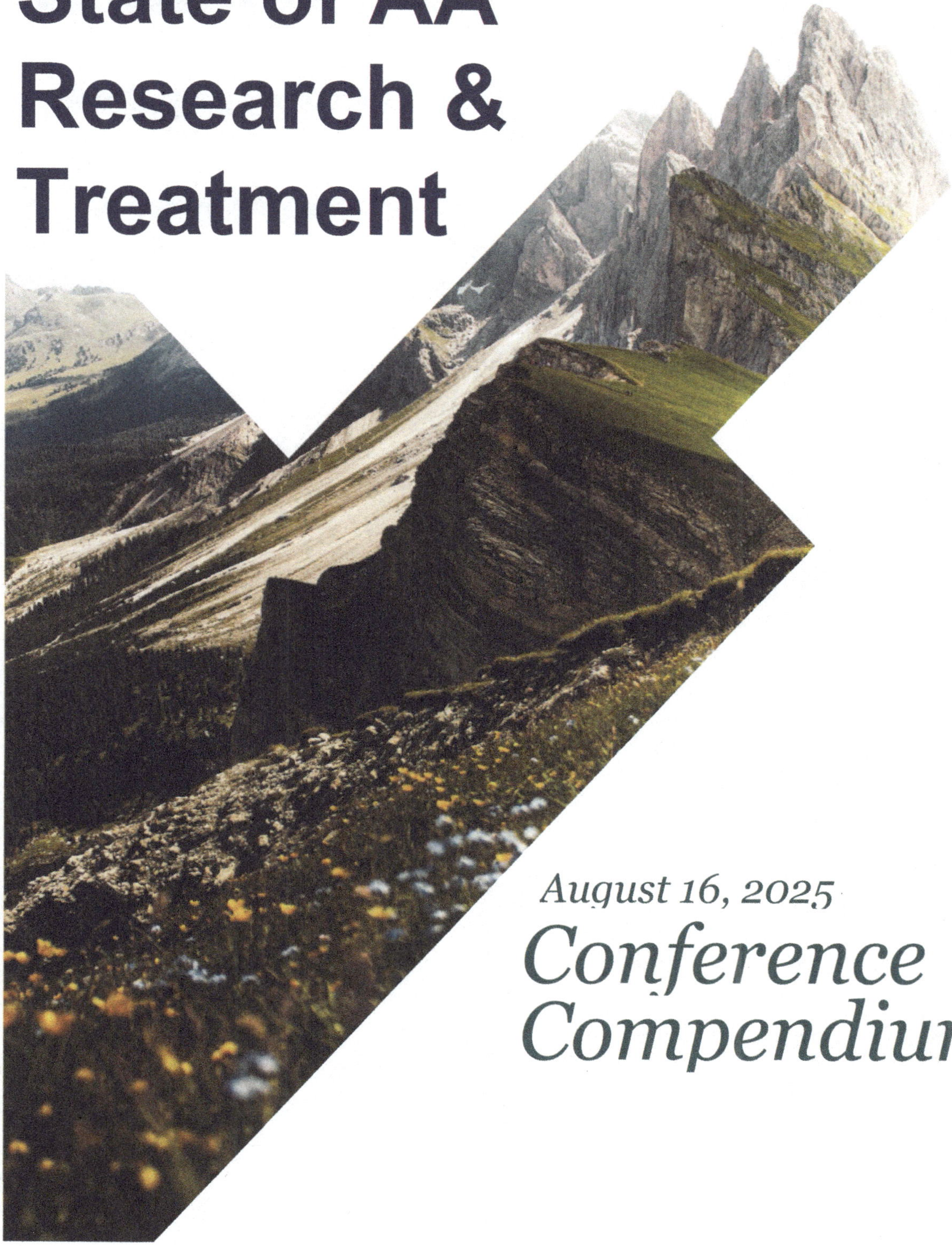

August 16, 2025

Conference Compendium

Introduction

State of Adhesive Arachnoiditis Research and Treatment Conference 2025

Westminster, Colorado USA
August 16, 2025

Co-Sponsored by:

Arachnoiditis Hope
Tennant Foundation and
Arachnoiditis and Chronic Meningitis Collaborative Research Network (ACMCRN)

Tennant Foundation
Arachnoiditis Hope
336 ½ S. Glendora Ave. West Covina, CA 91790
Tennantfoundation92@gmail.com

ACMCRN
Acmcrn.org

ISBN: 9781955934503
LOC: 2025918282
https:/doi.org/10.64611/cvwi6545

Conference Chairpersons and Organizers

Terri Anderson

Ingrid Hollis

Presenters

Forest Tennant, DrPH, MPH, MD

Martin J. Porcelli DO, PhD, MHPE, FACOFP

Evelyn Blackburn -VP Patient Engagement for ACMCRN

K Scott Guess PharmD, MS Pharm, RPh, APh

Amy Marx-Visual Artist

Dedication

We wish to gratefully thank all the tireless physicians, patient advocates, and family members who have paved the way for making this moment possible. Your work has not been in vain, as it has paved the way for this important conference to transpire in 2025.

Table of Contents

Introduction i

Conference Chairpersons and Organizers iii

Presenters iii

Dedication iii

Table of Contents v

Goals and Mission vii

What is an AA Educator and what does it mean? viii

Conference Agenda ix

Our Presenters: 1

Forest Tennant, DrPH, MPH, MD 2

Martin J. Porcelli DO, MHPE, FACOFP 3

Evelyn Blackburn VP Patient Engagement ACMCRN 4

K. Scott Guess PharmD, MSPharm, RPh, APh 5

Amy Marx 6

Presentations 7

Dr. Forest Tennant Presentation:State of AA Research and Treatment 2025: Dr. Forest Tennant 8

Clinical Treatment of AA: Dr. Martin Porcelli 40

Palliative Care for Advanced AA:Dr. Scott Guess 58

ACMCRN- One Team for Arachnoiditis: Advancing Research, Education, and Community: Evelyn Blackburn 74

Electro Medical Experience with Frequency Specific Microcurrents (FSM): Amy Marx 82

Appendix 85

Educational Document #2 87

Educational Document #25 88

Educational Document #32 89

Educational Document #48 90

Education Documents Index 91

Books by Dr. Forest Tennant: 93

Contact Information 94

Arachnoiditis Hope

State of Adhesive Arachnoiditis (AA) Research &Treatment Conference 2025

Goals and Mission

Arachnoiditis Hope Mission:

"Bring Diagnosis and Treatment of Adhesive Arachnoiditis (AA) to every Community."

Conference Mission:

To further the mission of Arachnoiditis Hope to "Bring Prevention, Diagnosis, and Treatment of Adhesive Arachnoiditis to Every Community."

Goals of Conference:

Develop a network of AA Educators

Establish Arachnoiditis and AA as a serious disease
Arachnoiditis and AA are serious diseases that need treatment

Build a foundation for research and study going forward

Adhesive Arachnoiditis (AA) Educator

What is an AA Educator and what does it mean?

·Counsel new patients

·Maintain referral sources

·Help facilitate research studies

·Advise troubled patients

·Sponsor education events

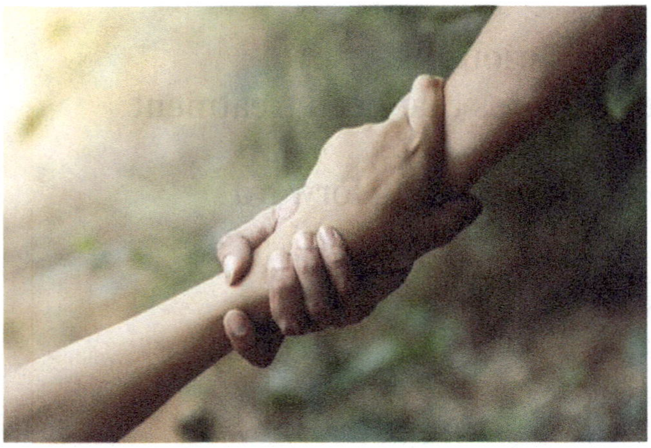

Conference Agenda

STATE OF AA RESEARCH AND TREATMENT
Co-Sponsored by Arachnoiditis Hope and
Arachnoiditis & Chronic Meningitis Collaborative Research Network
Marriott Westminster, 7000 Church Ranch Blvd,
Westminster, Colorado
Saturday, August 16, 2025

SATURDAY

6:30 - 8:30	Breakfast at Hotel (included in hotel rate-check with hotel when restaurant opens)
8:30 - 9:00	Registration
9:00 - 9:05	Welcome: Ingrid Hollis
9:05 - 11:00	Dr. Forest Tennant: State of AA Research and Treatment
11:00 - 11:15	Break
11:15 - 12:15	Dr. Martin Porcelli: Clinical Treatment of AA
12:15 - 1:45	Lunch on Your Own (Restaurants within Walking Distance)
1:45 - 2:30	Evelyn Blackburn ACMCRN: One Team for Arachnoiditis: Advancing Research, Education, and Community Together
2:30 - 3:30	Dr. Scott Guess Pharm D: Palliative Care for Advanced AA
3:30 - 3:45	Break
3:45 - 4:00	Amy Marx: Electro Medical Experience with Frequency Specific Microcurrent
4:00 - 4:30	Adhesive Arachnoiditis Patient Roundtable with Questions and Answers
4:30 - 5:00	Closing and Final Thoughts: Dr. Forest Tennant, Dr. Martin Porcelli, and Dr. Scott Guess
7PM	Dinner at Macaroni's Grill -Certificates presented

Our Presenters:

·Forest Tennant, DrPH, MPH, MD

·Martin J. Porcelli DO, MHPE, FACOFP

·K. Scott Guess PharmD, MSPharm, RPh, APh

·Evelyn Blackburn VP Patient Engagement ACMCRN

·Amy Marx

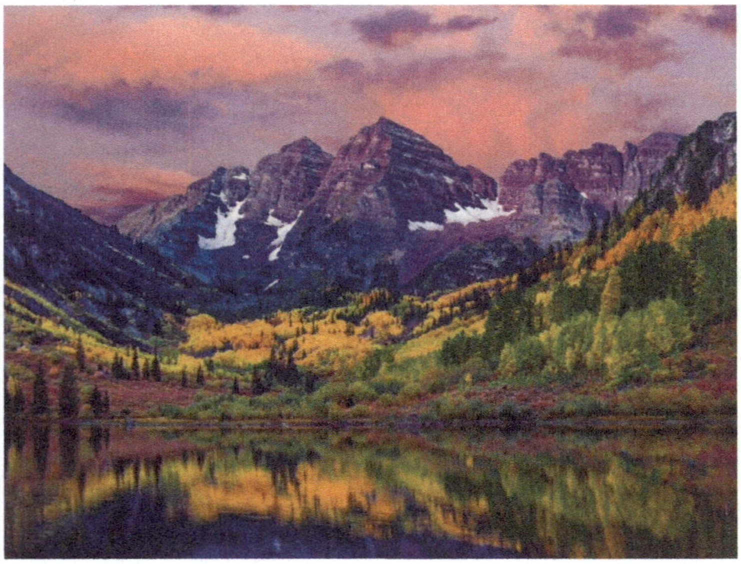

Forest Tennant, DrPH, MPH, MD

Biography:

Forest Tennant has spent most of his medical career as a practicing physician and researcher in the fields of addiction and pain medicine. He has published over 300 scientific articles and books in these fields. For his efforts he was recently given a "50 Year Achievement" award by "Pain Week". In this 50-year span he has been a US Army Medical Officer, UCLA Professor, Public Health Physician, Drug Advisor for the Los Angeles
Dodgers, NASCAR, and the National Football League. He was the editor of Practical Pain Management for 12 years. He recently retired from clinical practice to do research on intractable pain and the spinal cord disorder known as arachnoiditis. He and his wife, Miriam, have been married 59 years and they split their residence between West Covina, California and
Wichita, Kansas where they headquarter their real estate company, Tennant Homes. Their charitable giving and medical research are sponsored by the Tennant Foundation.

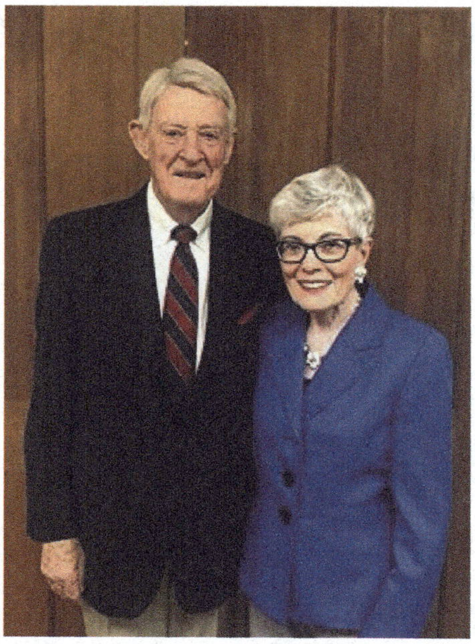

Dr. Forest Tennant and Mrs. Miriam Tennant

Martin J. Porcelli DO, MHPE, FACOFP

Dr. Porcelli is a Professor of Family Medicine at Western University of Health Sciences. He is also Assistant Professor of Family Medicine at UCLA School of Medicine.

Dr. Porcelli earned his Doctorate of Osteopathic Medicine degree at the Chicago College of Osteopathic Medicine in Illinois. He went back in the mid-80s and received his Master of Science in Education and his Doctor of Philosophy Degree in Business Management and Administration. He completed post graduate training at Tucson General Hospital and the University of Arizona School of Medicine in Tucson, AZ. He did further training/fellowship in Pain Management and Drug Addiction at West Center in Tucson, AZ.

Dr. Porcelli is certified and recertified in Family Medicine, Sports Medicine,
Geriatrics, Integrative Medicine, Osteopathic Manipulative Therapy, and Pain Management. He is a past President of the State Medical Society and two-time President of The Family Medicine Group in California.

He holds numerous elected positions at the American College of Osteopathic Family Physicians, The Education Research Foundation, and Emeritus position on the editorial board of The Journal of Southern California Clinicians, The American Osteopathic Association, and Osteopathic Family Physicians.

He has authored some 30 articles and is a frequent speaker for the Osteopathic profession, ACOFP, and AOA.

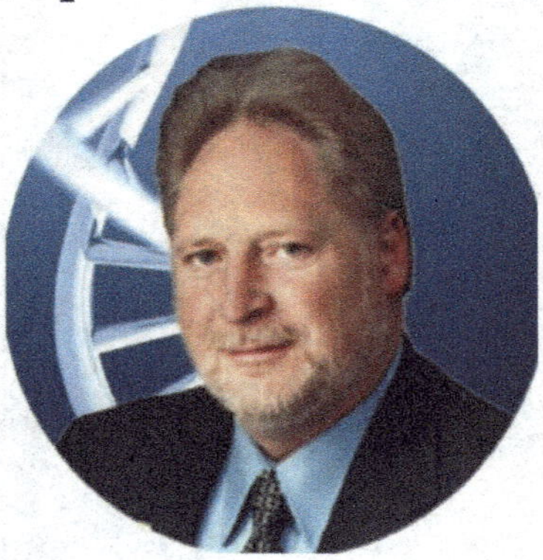

Dr. Martin J. Porcelli

Evelyn Blackburn VP Patient Engagement ACMCRN

Eve Blackburn is the Vice President of Patient Engagement at the Arachnoiditis & Chronic Meningitis Collaborative Research Network (ACMCRN). A catastrophic Adhesive Arachnoiditis patient and longtime advocate, Eve began her work as a Pain Patient Advocate in 2016 and joined ACMCRN in 2019. She leads the organization's patient engagement efforts and plays a key role in education, outreach, and infrastructure development. Eve also manages ACMCRN's website, social media, and graphic design, and created the curated physician list now used by patients worldwide.

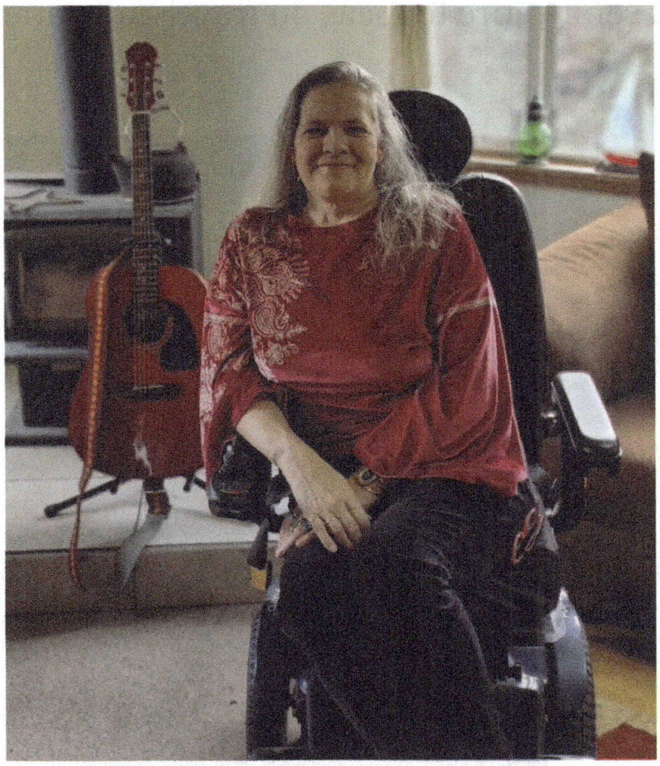

Eveyln Blackburn

K. Scott Guess PharmD, MSPharm, RPh, APh

Scott earned his Doctor of Pharmacy degree from the University of the Pacific in Stockton, California in 1983. He was beginning a career in chain retail pharmacy when he met Dr. Forrest Tennant. This began his journey in the field of Pain Management during which he opened his own pharmacies and attended the University of Florida to earn a Masters Degree in Pharmaceutical Outcomes Policy. A Masters Degree in Palliative Care from the University of Maryland followed. Dr. Guess was conferred the 42nd Advanced Practice Pharmacist Registration issued by California which allowed him to work as a physician extender seeing his own patients under the auspices of Dr. Tennant. Dr. Guess recently sold his pharmacy so he can semi-retire to focus on travel and patient advocacy.

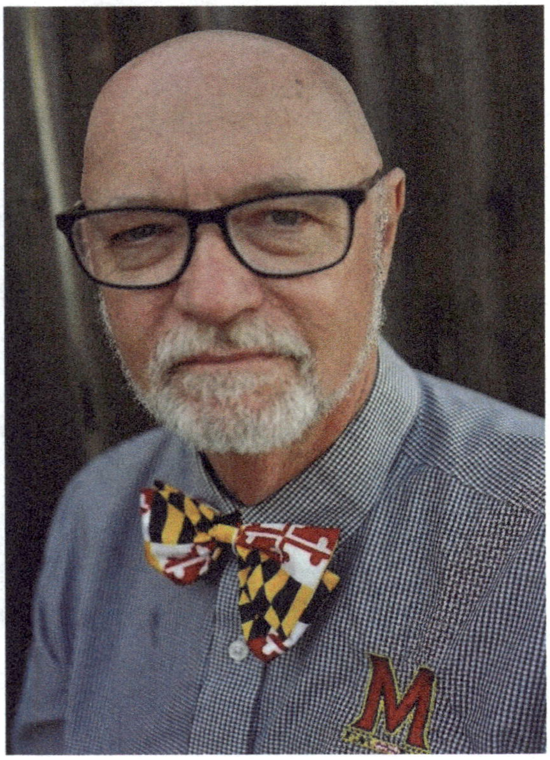

Dr. K. Scott Guess

Amy Marx

Amy Marx is an award-winning artist, custom jeweler, and real estate investor. Her oil paintings of storms and tornadoes have garnered significant attention in the press, on radio, and television, even appearing in a segment on the Weather Channel. She will be featured in the Women Artists of the DMV (DC, Maryland, Virginia) show, a 15-venue survey show of significant women artists of the region. Amy is also a real estate investor; renovating, renting and selling houses in Baltimore Maryland. Amy has found spiritual practices and development to have been of tremendous help in coping with the trauma of Adhesive Arachnoiditis. Seeing spiritual evolution as primary in our lives, she has pursued a number of different approaches. These have ranged from mediation to twelve-step programs to participating in The Pathwork for fifteen years and qualifying to be a teacher and trained to be a Pathwork Helper and following the tenants of Louise Hay, Abraham-Hicks and Unity Church. The underlying commonality and most important principles of which are that our thinking creates our lives and that, in order to heal one must both excavate the negative thought messages we are creating as a result of unhealed emotional trauma and then projecting into physical reality, and then change the message that we are thinking and projecting. She believes in a power greater than ourselves. She also believes that the work of this kind that she had done prior to the injury gave her an advantage in being able to both cope with and be led to the healing of it.

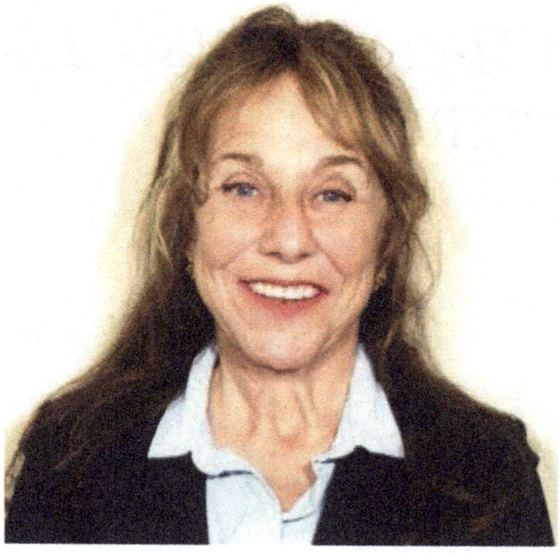

Amy Marx

Presentations

State of AA Research and Treatment 2025;

Dr. Forest Tennant

Clinical Treatment of AA;

Dr. Martin Porcelli

ACMCRN; One Team for Arachnoiditis: Advancing Research, Education, and Community Together;

Evelyn Blackburn

Palliative Care for Advanced AA;

Dr. Scott Guess

Electro Medical Experience with Frequency Specific Microcurrent;

Amy Marx

Dr. Forest Tennant Presentation:State of AA Research and Treatment 2025: Dr. Forest Tennant

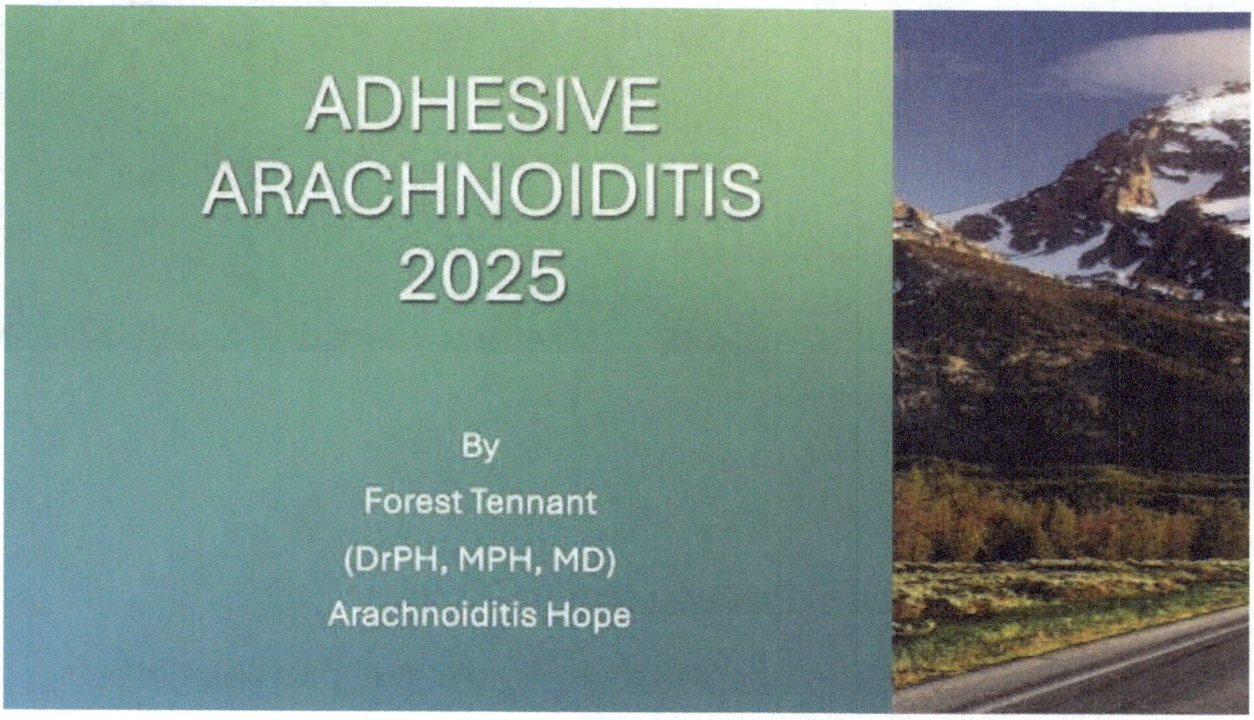

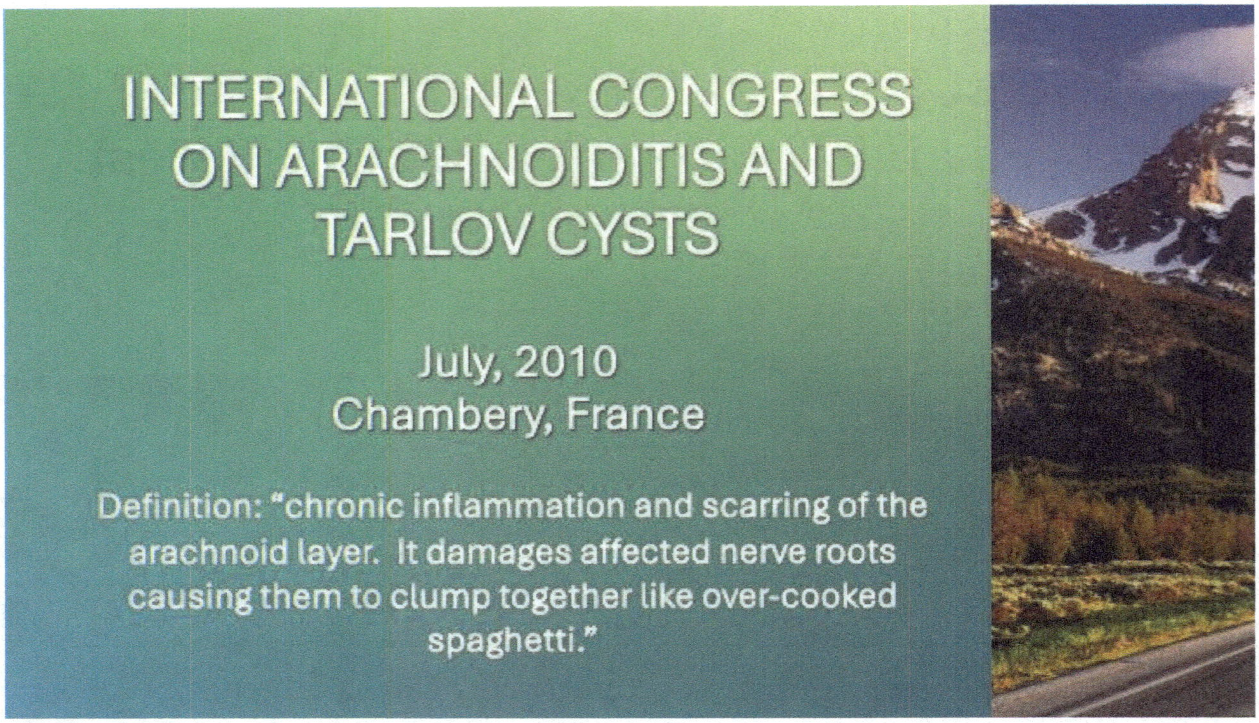

Definitions Used in Presentation

- Arachnoiditis – inflammation of the arachnoid membrane, major clinical problem areas are the cervical and lumbar spines
- Adhesive arachnoiditis – a chronic inflammatory disease in which cauda equina nerve roots become adhered to the arachnoid membrane by adhesions
- Autoimmunity – process in which a biologic element erroneously recognizes normal tissue as foreign and attacks the tissue producing inflammation and tissue destruction
- Genetic connective tissue disease – a heritable condition in which collagen in tissue is deficient in quantity or quality producing weakness and deterioration. Most common is Ehlers-Danlos Syndrome.

Two Basic Causes

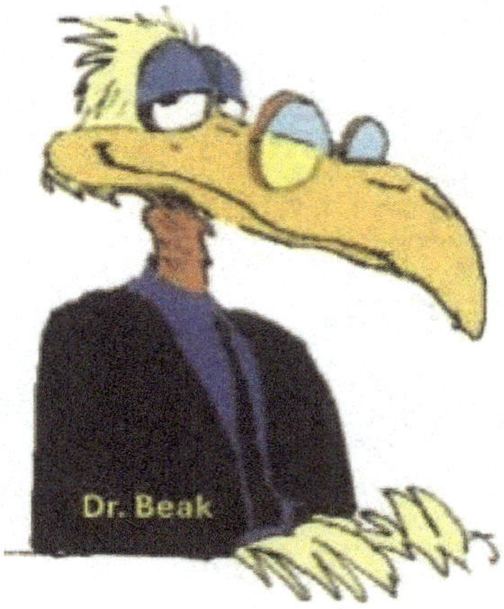

1. Direct trauma to the spine (examples: vehicular accident, fall, electrocution)

2. Inflammatory/autoimmune process that may originate outside the spine or develop within the spine

Prevalence and Incidence – Seemingly Increasing

✓Still classified as a rare or unusual disease

✓MRI technology and recognition

✓Spinal medical interventions (i.e., epidural injections)

✓Viral infections and reactivations

✓Degenerative disc disease in young adults

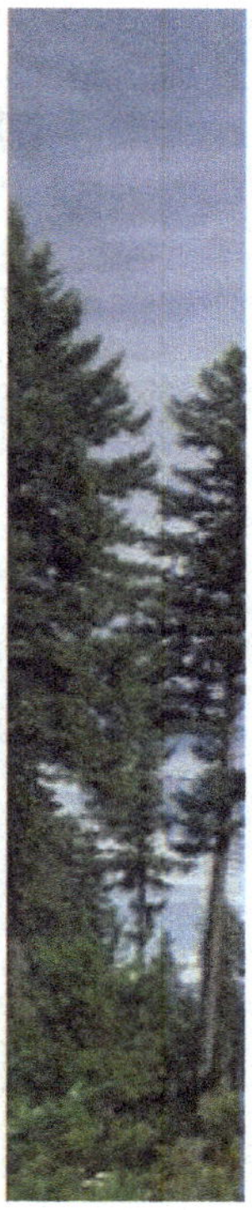

Clinical Profile of 80 MRI-Documented Cases of AA

Demographic Factor	Number (%)
Females	65 (81%)
Males	15 (19%)
Age range in years	18 to 80
Mean age ± S.D. in years	48.9 ± 13.7
Predisposing spinal conditions*	61 (76.3%)
Herniated discs	44 (55%)
Spondylolisthesis	17 (21.25%)
Osteoporosis	6 (7.5%)
Spine arthritis	23 (28.75%)
Scoliosis	9 (11.25%)
Tarlov cysts	9 (11.25%)

Prior Surgeries and Injections

Demographic Factor	Number (%)
One or more spinal surgeries	43 (53.8%)
Total No. of spine surgeries in 43 cases	91
Range of surgeries in 43 cases	1 to 8
No. who had 2 or more spine surgeries	22 (27.5%)
No. who had 1 or more epidural injections	69 (86.3%)
Total No. epidural injections in 69 cases	236
Range of epidural injection in 69 cases	1 to 20
No. reported over 8 epidural injections	16 (20%)

Complications Reported by Over 55% of Cases

Demographic Factor	Number (%)
Pain relief on standing	70 (87.5%)
Standing too long causes need to lie down	69 (86.3%)
Hurts to lie flat on back	67 (83.8%)
Pain always present	66 (82.5%)
Shooting pains, tremors, or jerking in legs	64 (80%)
Burning pains in feet	63 (78.8%)
Cold hands or feet	58 (72.5%)
Crawling insects on skin	58 (72.5%)
Water dripping down legs	53 (66.3%)
Difficulty starting urination/defecation	51 (63.8%)
Leg raising hurts back	50 (62.5%)
Blurred vision	47 (58.8%)
Pain behind eyes	45 (56.3%)

Risk Factors and Predisposing Conditions

✓Herniated, "slipped" disc

✓Genetic connective tissue disease (i.e., Ehlers-Danlos Syndrome)

✓Anatomic spine abnormality (i.e., scoliosis)

✓Autoimmune disease (i.e., psoriasis, ankylosing spondylitis)

✓Severe infection (i.e., Lyme, meningitis, covid, pneumonia)

✓Spinal medical procedure (i.e., epidural injection)

✓Infectious mononucleosis

✓Multi-system disease (2 or more painful conditions)

✓Severe Trauma

The Pathologic Process

Inflammation must simultaneously develop in both the arachnoid membrane (inner lining of the spinal canal cover) and cauda equina nerve roots. The inflammation must progress to a stage that adhesions fuse (glue) the two tissues together to form a mass that entraps cauda equina nerve roots.

A Catastrophic Event!

Normal Spine

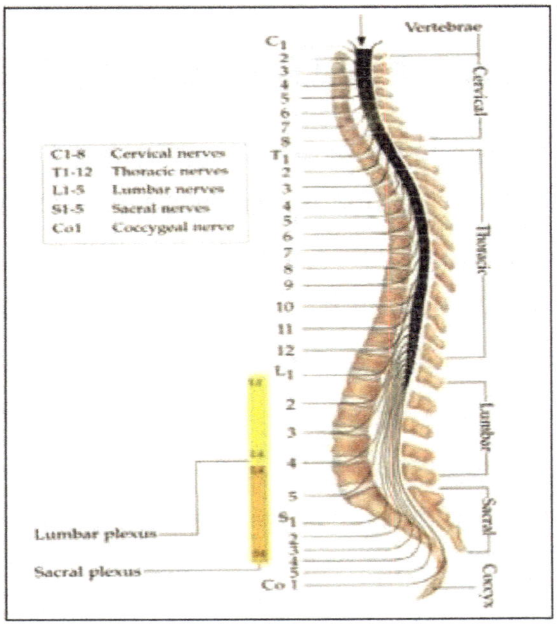

11

Basic Anatomy of the Lumbar-Sacral Spine

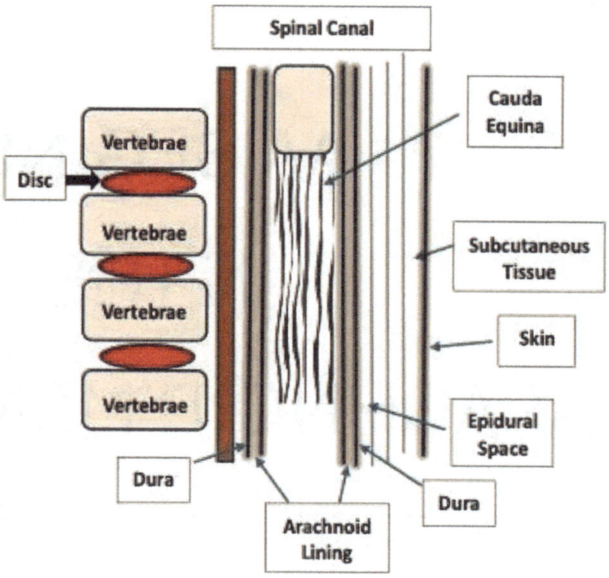

Definition of Arachnoid

The arachnoid membrane often called arachnoid is the inner layer or lining of the spinal canal cover. The outer layer is the dura.

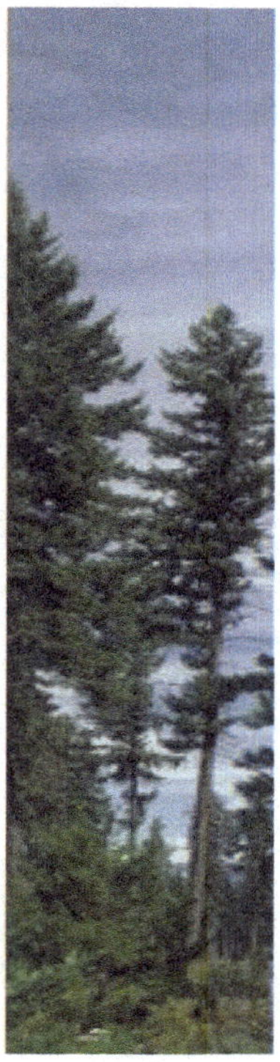

AA BEGINS
IN THE
ARACHNOID MEMBRANE

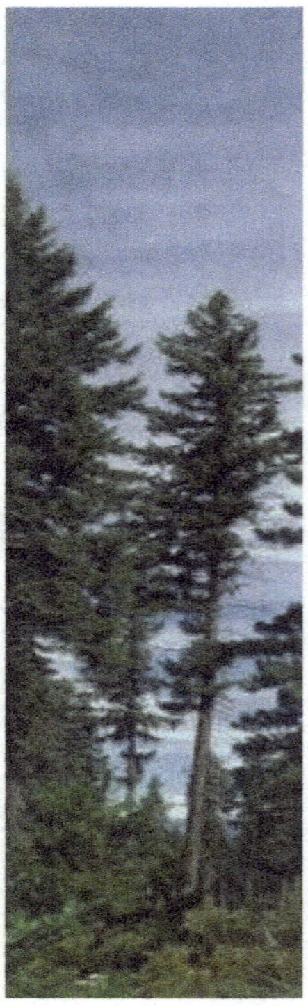

14

<u>Biologic Functions of the Arachnoid</u>

1. Protective lining of canal cover (dura)

2. Spinal fluid transfer to lymph and blood

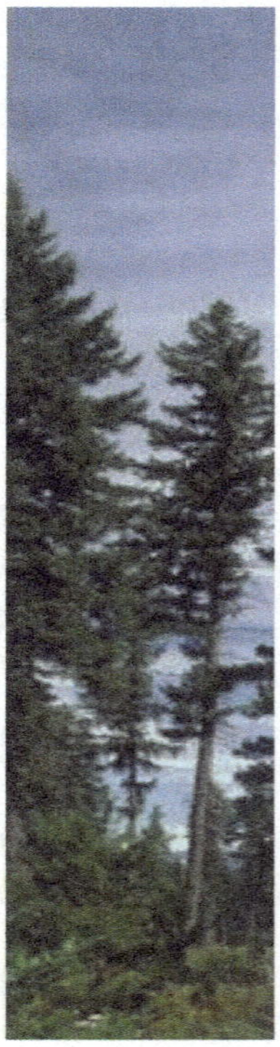

15

Some Biologic Characteristics

- Has no blood supply or nerves
- Soft-composed of collagen and fibroblasts
- Only cell surface tolerates spinal fluid

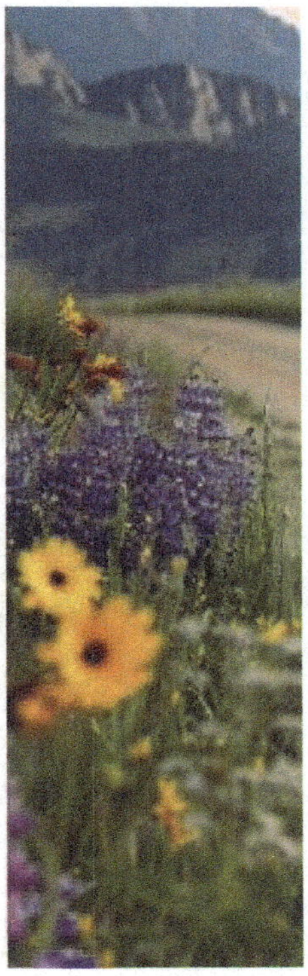

Electron Microscopic Picture of Arachnoid

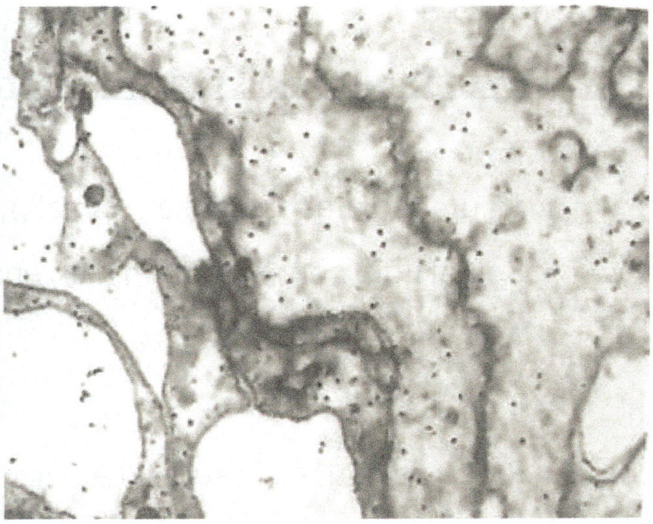

Electron Microscopy X 40,000

The Cells of the Arachnoid

The Arachnoid Membrane Head-On View

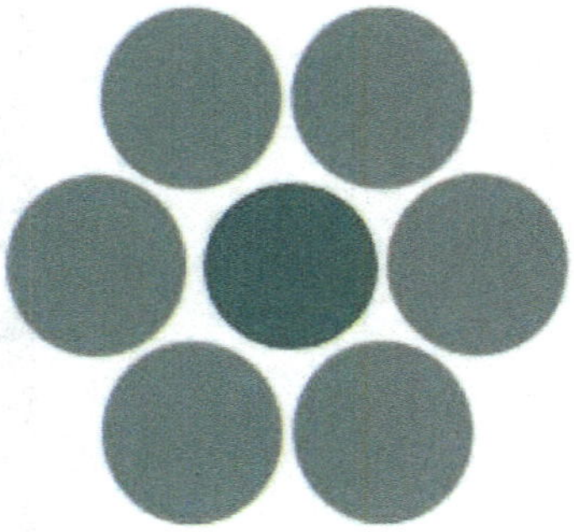

About 10 Layers Deep

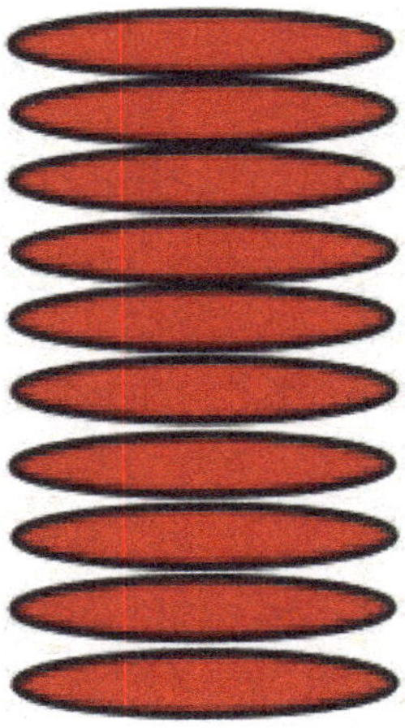

How Inflammation Originates in the Arachnoid Membrane

- ✓Trauma to arachnoid (i.e., spinal puncture)
- ✓Spinal fluid contamination (i.e., epidural injection)
- ✓Autoimmunity
- ✓Infection
- ✓Pressure causes fissures (i.e., disc, epidural fluid)

Easy Target for Disease

- ✓Soft-easily cracked or fissured
- ✓Invasion by virus or bacteria
- ✓Inflammation poorly controlled
- ✓Connective tissue disorder (EDS) – weak tissue
- ✓May disconnect from dura (Tarlov cysts)
- ✓Spreads inflammation to dura and cauda equina
- ✓Causes seepage and leaks

20

Needle Puncture

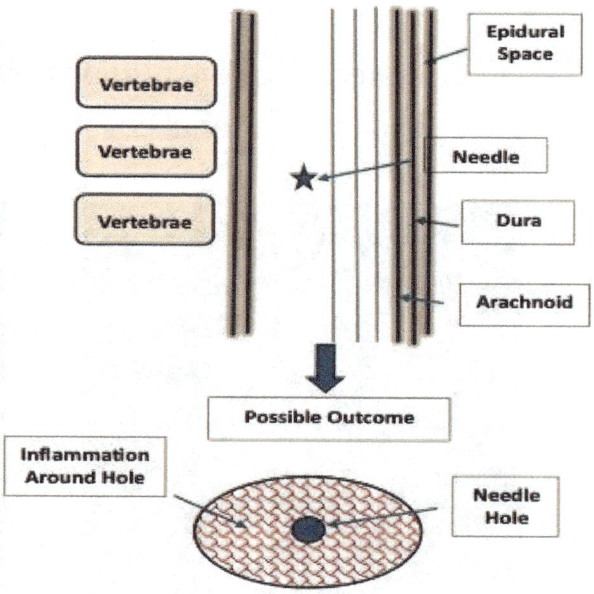

Epidural Pressure by Disc or Fluid Can Fissure Arachnoid

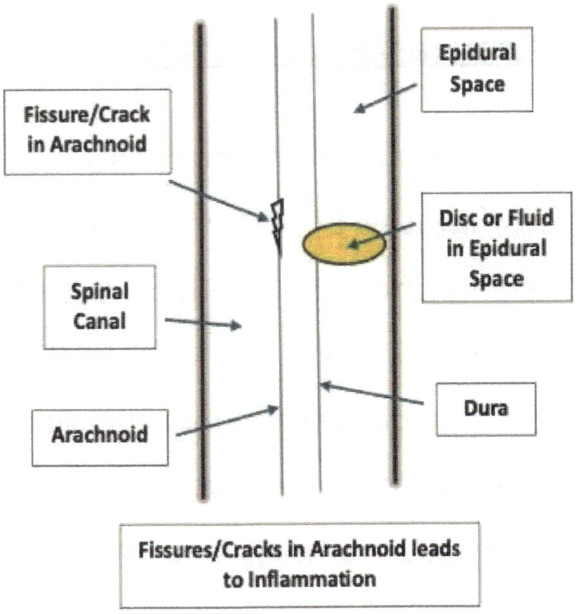

Degenerated discs are putting pressure on the dura and arachnoid (spinal canal cover)

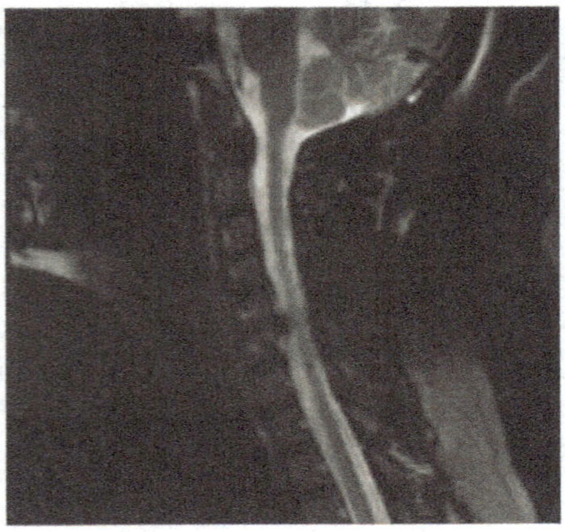

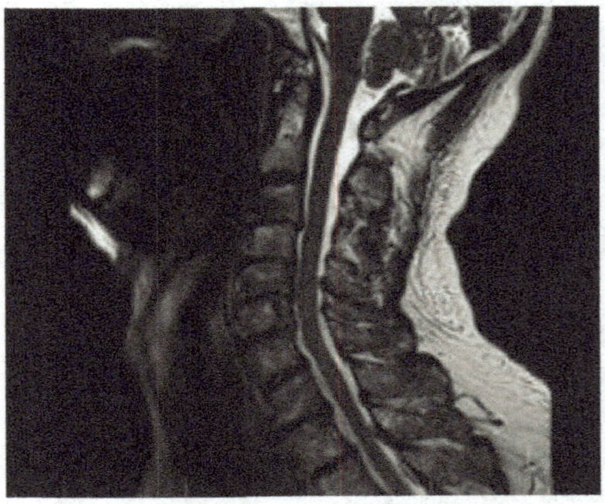

Degenerated discs are pressing on the spinal canal.

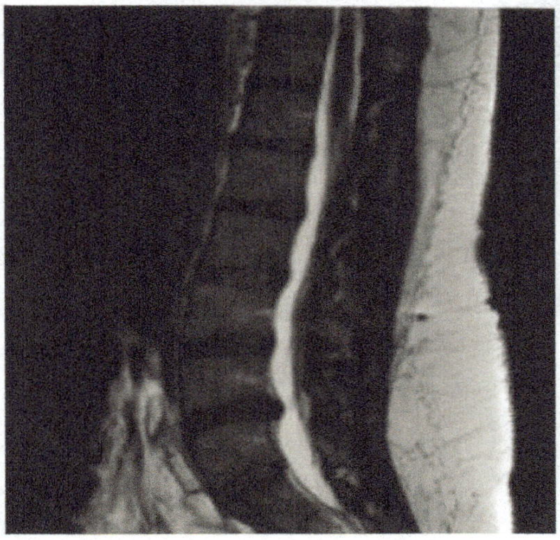

Adhesive arachnoiditis is on the right side.

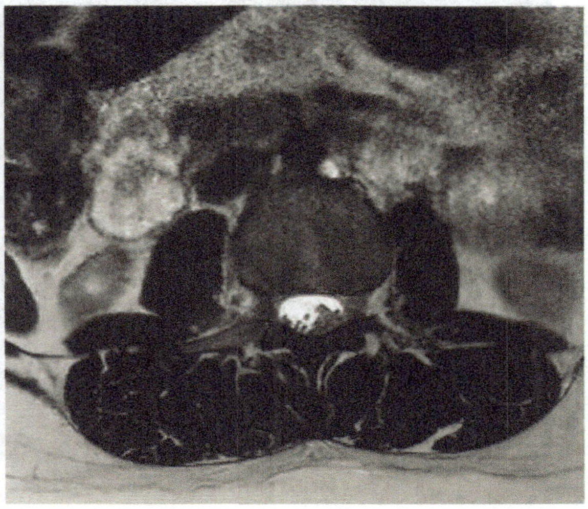

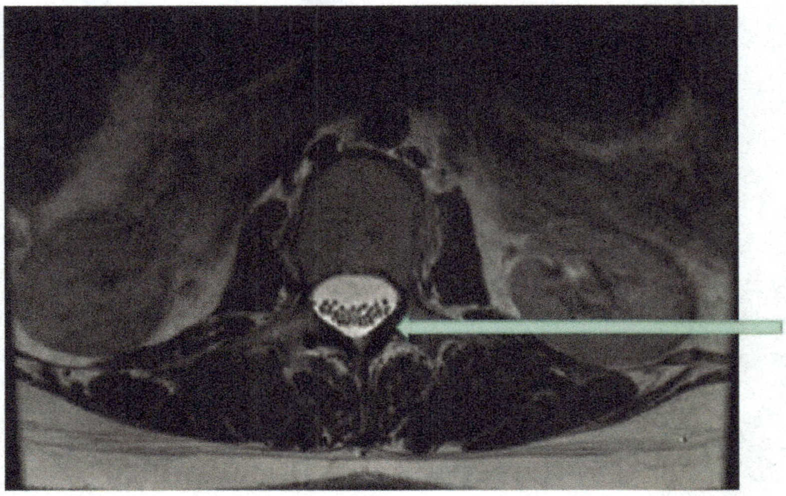

Canal cover thickened on this side compared to the opposite side

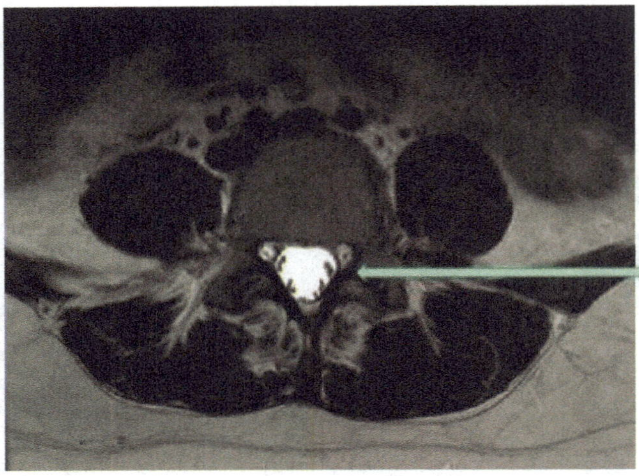

Right spinal cover thickened compared to the opposite side

Arachnoid Injury to AA

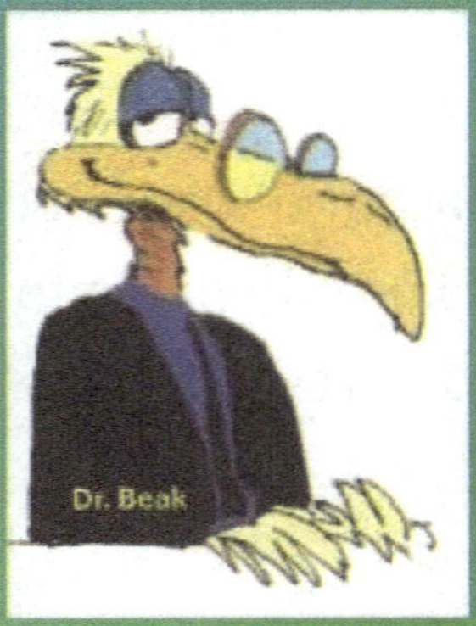

Hole or Fissure

↓

Inflammation Around Site

↓

Acute ARC

↓

Chronic ARC

↓

Adhesive Arachnoiditis

Spinal Fluid Leak

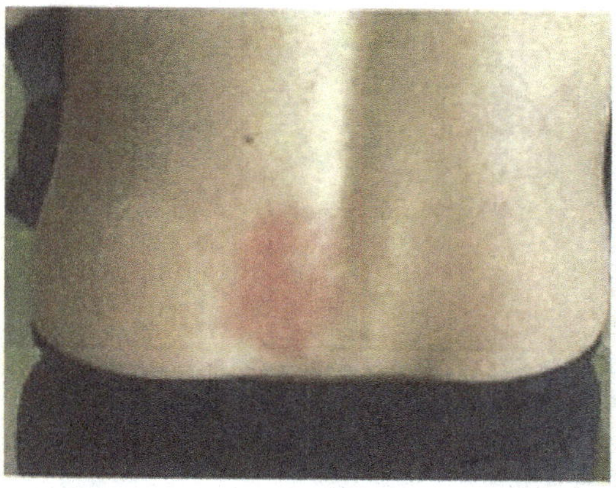

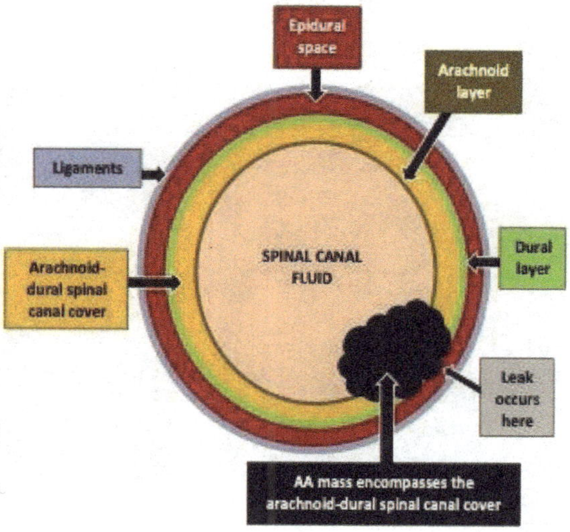

[28]

Diagnosis

Eight major symptoms, four or more are diagnostic

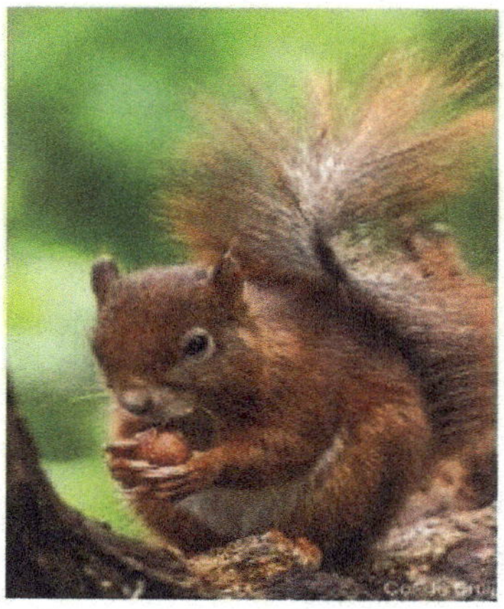

1	Sharp, stabbing pains in your lower back, buttocks, or groin/crotch area when you twist, turn, or bend
2	Bizarre skin sensations such as crawling insects or water dripping down one or both legs
3	Burning pains in your feet and/or groin/crotch area
4	Your pain temporarily lessens when you stand or recline
5	Leg weakness
6	Pain that radiates down one or both legs
7	Bladder dysfunction that may include dribbling, urgency, or difficulty stating or stopping urination
8	Head or cerebral symptoms which may include headache, vertigo, dizziness, or blurred vision

AA Produces Indentations and Contractures

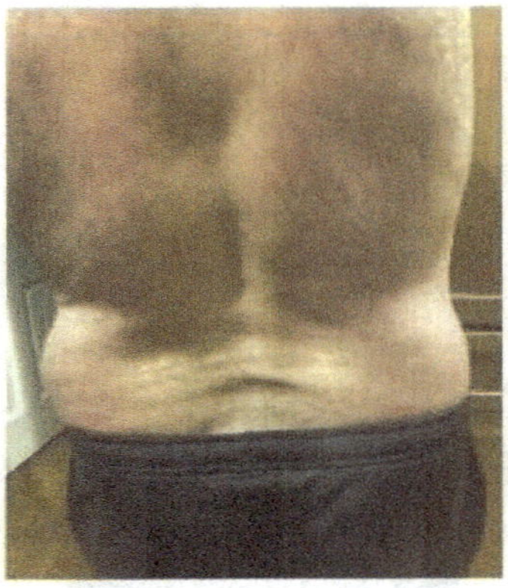 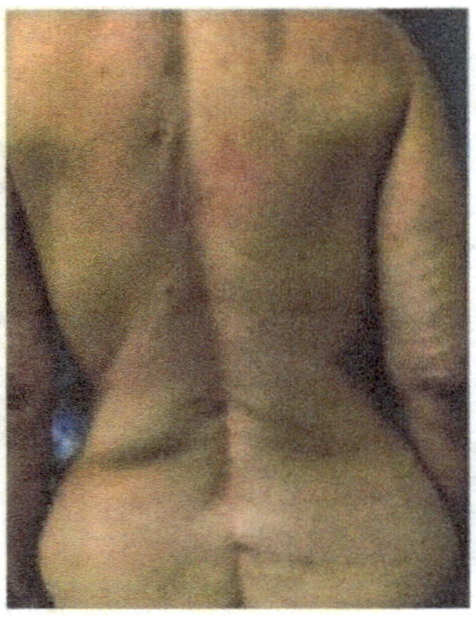 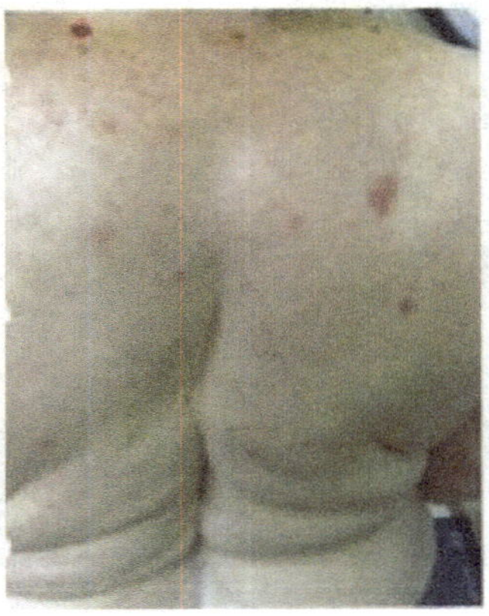

30

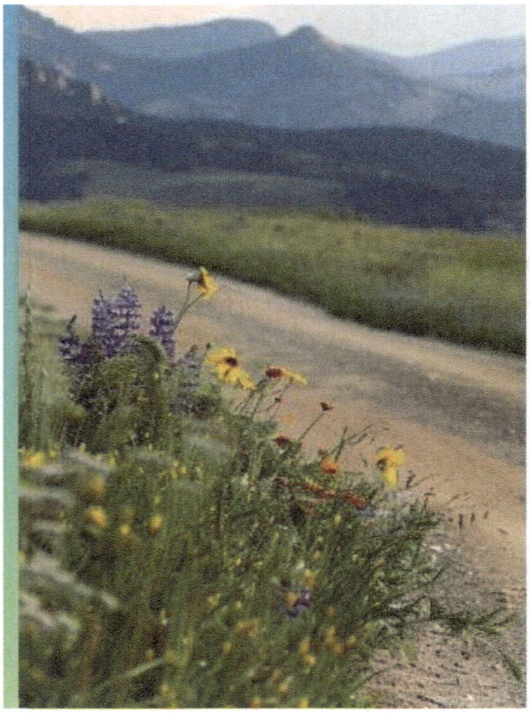

MRI Confirmation

✓Classic – nerve root clumping with attachment to arachnoid

✓Peripheralization of nerve roots (empty sac)

Examples of Adhesive Arachnoiditis

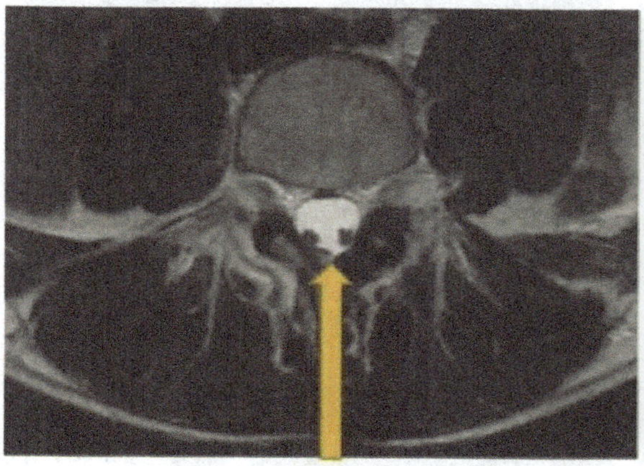

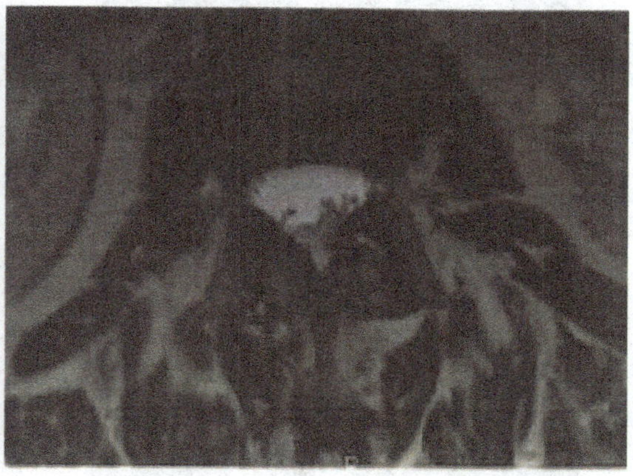

[32]

Examples of Peripheralization

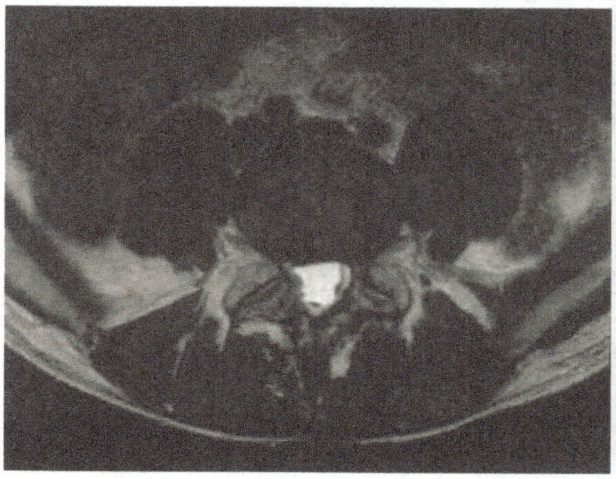

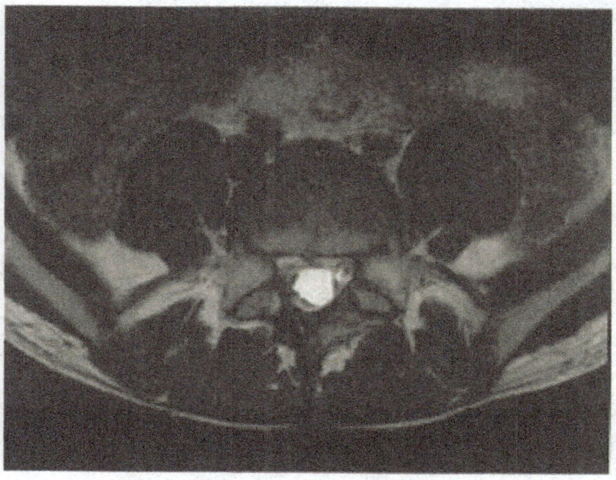

[31]

Empty Sac **Tarlov Cyst**

Typical findings in Ehlers-Danlos Syndrome

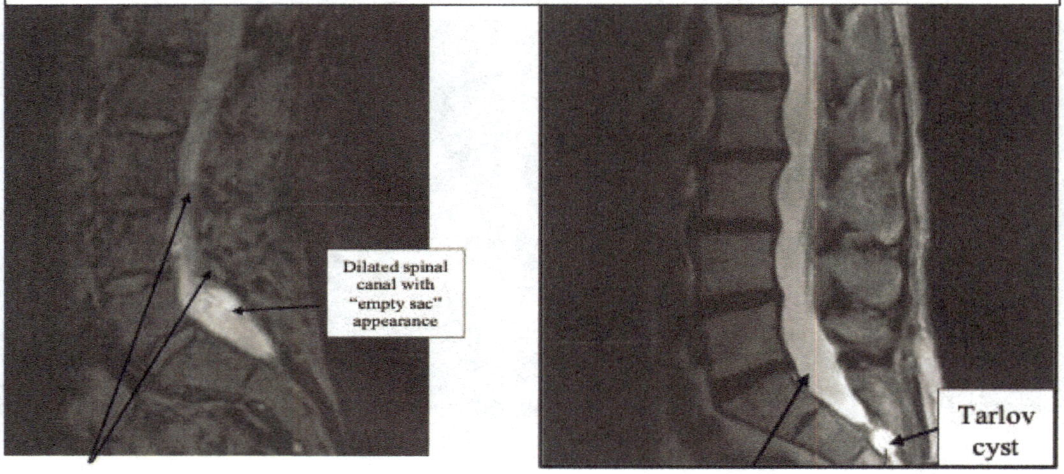

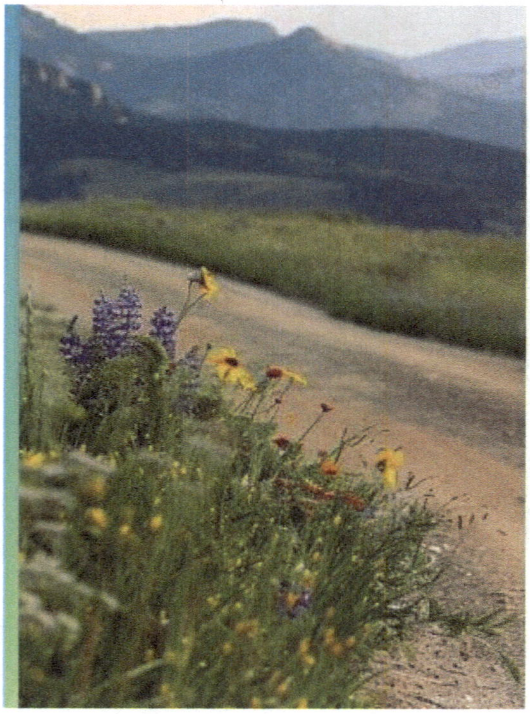

Emergency Treatment Options

Emergency Option 1:

Intravenous methylprednisolone 100 to 500 mg daily for 3 to 5 days.

Emergency Option 2:

1. Ketorolac (Toradol®) 30 to 60 mg (injection) once a day for 3 consecutive days.
2. Medrol® (methylprednisolone) 6-Day Dose Pak.
3. Medroxyprogesterone 10 mg 2 times a day for 3 to 5 days.

Three-Component Treatment

CONTROL Suppression of Inflammation	CURATIVE Regeneration of Damaged Tissue	SYMPTOMATIC Control of Pain
Direct suppression Viral control	Neuroregeneration	Ascending – Descending Neuropathic
	Dissolution of Adhesions	

Suppression of Inflammation

Prescription Medicinals	Non-Prescription Medicinals	Our 1st Choice
Diclofenac Dexamethasone Methylprednisolone Ketorolac	Serrapeptase Curcumin/Turmeric Astragalus Luteolin Quercetin	Low dose ketorolac And Methylprednisolone

Basic Protocol

Summary: A short-acting opioid plus low dose ketorolac and methylprednisolone.

1. Pain Relief: A short-acting opioid taken only as needed.

a. Tramadol (Ultram®), 50 – 100 mg
b. Codeine/acetaminophen, 30 – 60 mg
c. Buprenorphine, 2 – 4 mg
d. Hydrocodone (Vicodin®, Norco®), 10 mg
e. Oxycodone (Percocet®), 5 – 10 mg

2. Low Dose Ketorolac and Methylprednisolone

a. Ketorolac PO, 10 mg twice a day on Monday/Thursday. Option: Injection of 15 to 30 mg on Monday/Thursday.
b. Methylprednisolone 4 mg PO on Tuesday/Friday

Why Methylprednisolone?

Bibliography on Spine

Bibliography on Methylplrednisolone on Spinal Cord Inflammation and Injury

1. Bracken MB, Shepard MJ, Thorpe K, et al. A randomized, controlled trial of methylprednisolone or naltrexone in the treatment of acute spinal cord injury: results of the Second National Acute Spinal Cord Injury Study. *N Engl J Med* 1990;322:1405-1411.
2. Bracken MB, Shepard MJ, Holfor TR, et al. Administration of methylprednisolone for 24 or 48 hours of tirilazad mesylate for 48 hours in the treatment of acute spinal cord injury: results of the Third National Acute Spinal Canal Injury Randomized Controlled Trial. *JAMA* 1997;277:1597-1604.
3. Hall ED, Braughler JM. Effects of intravenous methylprednisolone on spinal cord lipid peroxidation and (Na',K)-ATPase activity: dose response analysis during 1st hour after contusion injury in the cat. *J Neurosurg* 1982;49:563-568.
4. Chikawa T, Ikata T, Katoh S, et al. Preventive effects of lecithinized superoxide dismutase and methylprednisolone on spinal cord injury in rats: transcriptional regulation of inflammatory and neurotrophic genes. *J Neurotrauma* 2001;18:93-103.
5. Bartholdi D, Schwab ME. Methylprednisolone inhibits early inflammatory processes but not ischemic cell death after spinal cord lesion in the rat. *Brain Res* 1995;672:177-182.
6. Ku J, Fan G, Chen S. et al. Methylprednisolone inhibition of TNF-(alpha) expression and NF-kappaB activation after spinal cord injury in rats. *Brain Res Mol Brain Res* 1998;59:135-142.
7. Kumida M, Inaba H, Isawa E, et al. Prevention by methylprednisolone of increased circulating tumor necrosis factor-alpha levels and lung injury associated with systemic inflammatory response syndrome due to intraperitoneal hyperthermia. *Anesth Analog* 1999;88:771-776.
8. Rabchevsky AG, Fugaccia I, Sullivan PG, et al. Efficacy of methylprednisolone therapy for the injured rat spinal cord. *J Neurosci Res* 2002;68:7-18.
9. Fu ES, Saporta S. Methylprednisolone inhibits production of interleukin-1 beta and interleukin-6 in the spinal cord following compression injury in rats. *J Neurosurg Anesth* 2005;17:82-85.

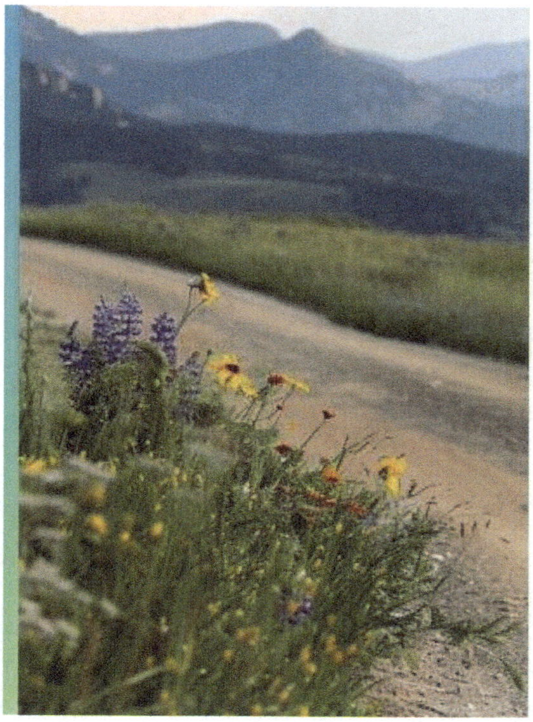

Flare Treatment

✓6-Day Medrol® Dose Pak

Options:

Methylprednisolone, 10-20 mg injection with or without

Ketorolac 30mg

Regeneration of Tissues (Neuroregeneration)

Peptides	Hormones	Our 1st Choice
BPC-157 Thymosin KPV ARA 290	Palmitoylethanolamide (PEA) DHEA HCG Colostrum Medroxyprogesterone Nandrolone Whole adrenal	Palmitoylethanolamide (PEA) with BPC-157

Dissolution of Adhesions

Medicinals	Electromedical
Pentoxifylline Vitamin E Serrapeptase Nattokinase	Microcurrent Laser Radio frequency

Control of Pain

Ascending	Descending	Neuropathic
Low dose naltrexone, opioids, ketamine, PEA, marijuana, CBD	Methylphenidate, amphetamine salts (Adderall®), dextroamphetamine, phentermine, modafinil, tizanidine, clonidine, lion's mane, St. John's wort	Diazepam (Valium®), carisoprodol (Soma®), Lorazepam (Ativan®), Triazolam (Xanax®), gabapentin, baclofen, KAVA
Electrical stimulators and intrathecal pumps may be required.		

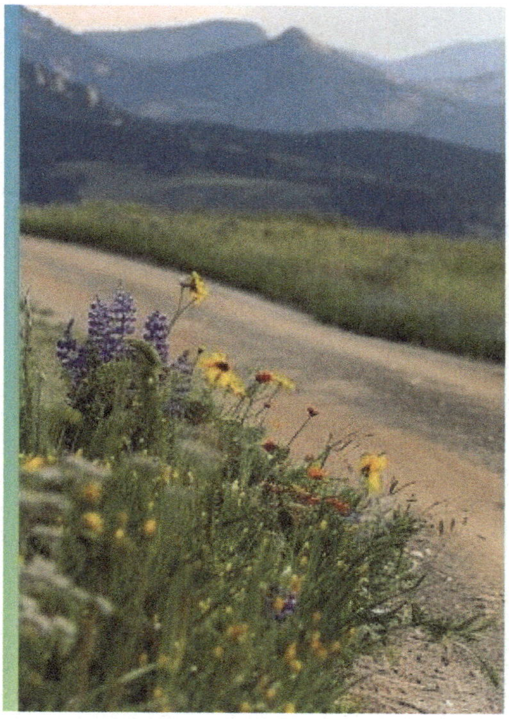

Ultra High Potency Hydromorphone

An alternative to stimulators and pumps in persons who fail standard pain treatment. A 0.1 to 0.2 ml of 50 mg.ml hydromorphone is subcutaneously injected with an insulin or allergy syringe.

Anazao Laboratories
5710 Hoover Blvd.
Tampa, FL 33634
Ph: 1-888-280-4331
Website: www.anazaohealth.com

Treatment Support Measures

✓Daily Protein Anti-Inflammatory Diet

✓Spinal Fluid Flow Exercises

✓Exercises for Strength and Paralysis Prevention

46

Epstein-Barr Virus Reactivation – Causative Factor

Our studies continue to indicate it is a causative factor in multi-system disease and adhesive arachnoiditis.

Key Point: Painful conditions require an ongoing generator of inflammation to produce pain and physiologic impairments.

47

Epstein-Barr Virus (EBV) Antibodies in 110 Patients With Adhesive Arachnoiditis				
		No. Tested	No. + Positive	%
1	EBV Viral Capsid IgG Antibody (VCA)	106	105	99.1
2	EBV Nuclear Antigen IgG Antibody (EBNA)	105	99	94.3
3	EBV Viral Capsid IgM Antibody (VCA IgM)	94	5	5.3
4	Early Nuclear Antigen IgG Antibody (EA-EBNA IgG)	41	29	70.7

Problems with EBV

Reactivation may leave behind

- Autoimmunity
- Chronic tissue infiltration
- Partner with Lyme and other viruses

Characteristics of Reactivation

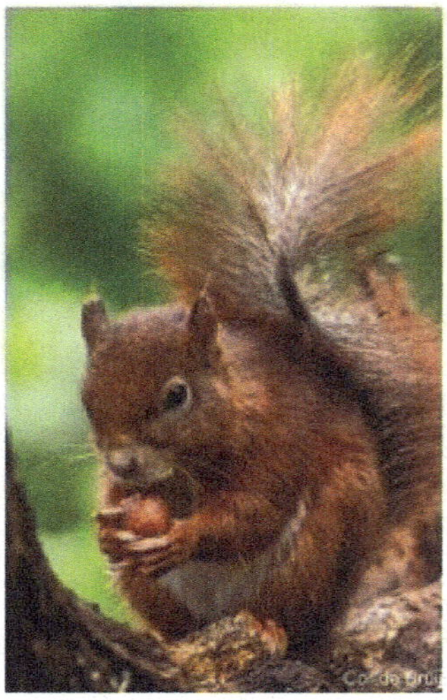

- Asymptomatic autoimmunity and/or tissue invasion
- Cause of multi-system disease
- Specific cancers, 1.5 to 2% of the world's cancers
- Proclivity for neuronal tissue

Painful Conditions That Preceded Adhesive Arachnoiditis in Patients With Elevated EBV Antibodies N = 36		
CONDITION	No.	%
Arthritis	36	100
Neuropathies	36	100
Herniated discs	29	80.5
Migraine	27	75
Fibromyalgia	22	61.1
Irritable bowel	21	58.3
Temporal mandibular joint (TMJ)	20	55.6
Tarlov cyst	18	50.0
Bursitis	18	50.0
Sciatica	17	47.2
Loss of teeth	17	47.2
Spinal fluid leaks	15	41.7
Plantar fasciitis	15	41.7
Tendonitis	13	36.1
Complex regional pain syndrome (CRPS)	9	25.0
Costochondritis	8	22.2

Reactivation Takes Place When the Body is Temporarily Immune Deficient

- Accident
- Trauma
- Infection
- Psychologic

Two Kinds of Autoimmunity

1. Autoantibodies

2. Cellular Mimicry

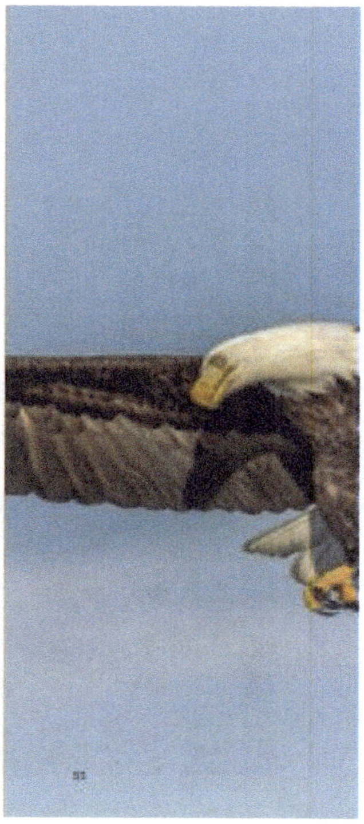

Two Pathologic Concerns in Persons with AA

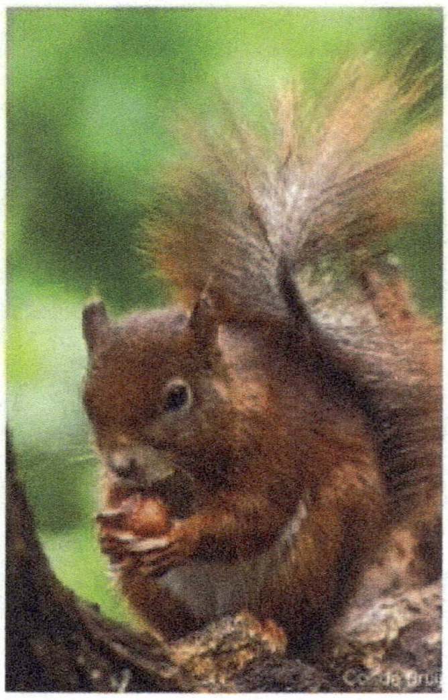

1. Two major antibodies are 2 times normal, viral capsid (VCA), nuclear antigen (EBNA). Virus not reactivated.
2. Both major antibodies are elevated, and virus has reactivated. Indicative tests are:

- Early VCA – positive
- Polymer Chain Reaction (DNA) - positive

Prevention of Reactivation

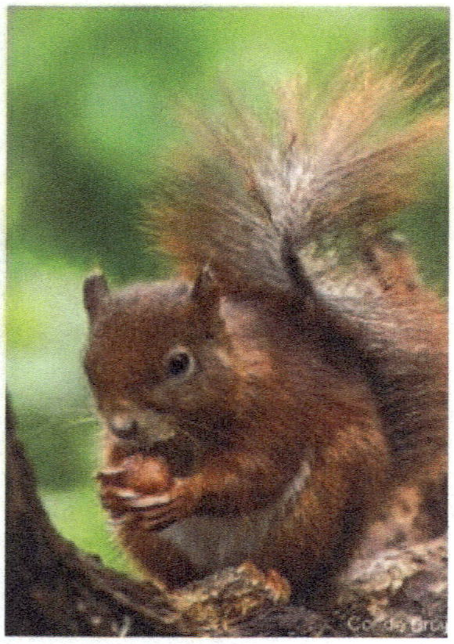

1. Critical vitamins/minerals
2. Medicinals for prevention of reactivation
    a. Andrographis
    b. Luteolin
    c. Curcumin
    d. Astragalus

Critical Vitamins and Minerals

A person with AA is well advised to use more than one mineral. Take one of the minerals each day. They can be rotated.

- Vitamin C, 2000 mg in AM and PM
- Vitamin B-12, 500 to 1000 mcg daily
- Vitamin D, 500 to 800 units a day
- Minerals: magnesium, selenium, zinc, boron

Measures for Elevated Antibodies But No Reactivation

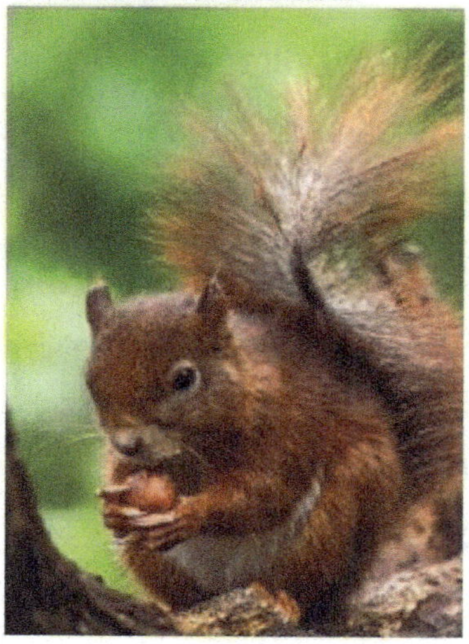

Suppressive Agents

1. Monolaurin
2. Thymosin

Option: Elimination Agent

Ivermectin – short trial

Protective Agents

Ketorolac and methylprednisolone

Options for Reactivation

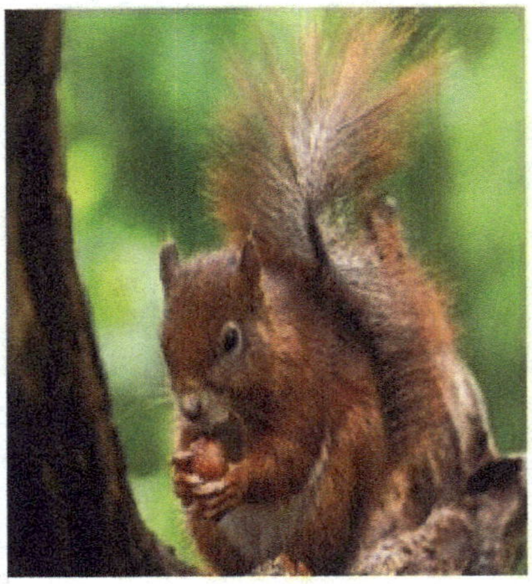

1. Antiviral agents:
   a. acyclovir
   b. valacyclovir
2. Lysine
3. Ivermectin
4. Prednisone

In addition to the above preventive measures to prevent reactivation and monolaurin is recommended.

The Ehlers-Danlos Syndrome Connection

EDS is a heritable connective tissue disease in which collagen quantity and quality are deficient. EDS frequently causes multi-system disease. Intervertebral discs and the arachnoid membrane are high collagen concentration tissues that are subject to EDS deterioration. EDS is a known immune deficiency disease. Infections including EBV are common. For treatment and prevention of AA, we recommend aggressive anabolic, neuroregeneration measures including diet, hormones, and peptides.

Tarlov Cyst – AA Connection

A cyst inside the spinal canal is a "bubble" or outpouching of the arachnoid membrane. Cysts are common with EDS. The arachnoid membrane in and around the cyst is defective and prone to inflammation. We recommend inflammatory prophylaxis and anabolic measures to prevent AA.

[60]

Areas of Ongoing Research

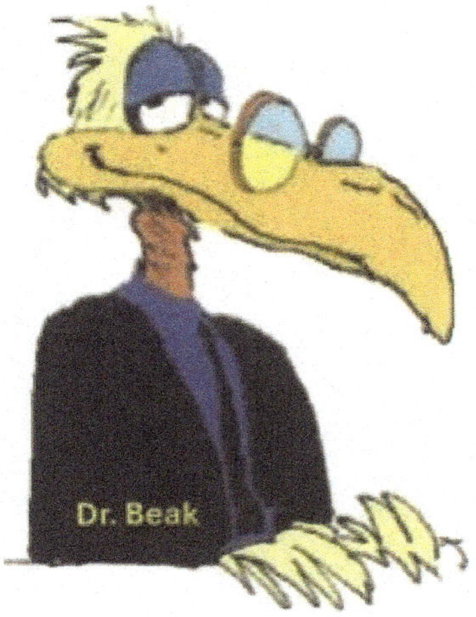

- Stem Cells
- Electromedical
- Microsurgery
- Viral Reactivation
- Radiation
- Neuroregeneration

[61]

Clinical Treatment of AA: Dr. Martin Porcelli

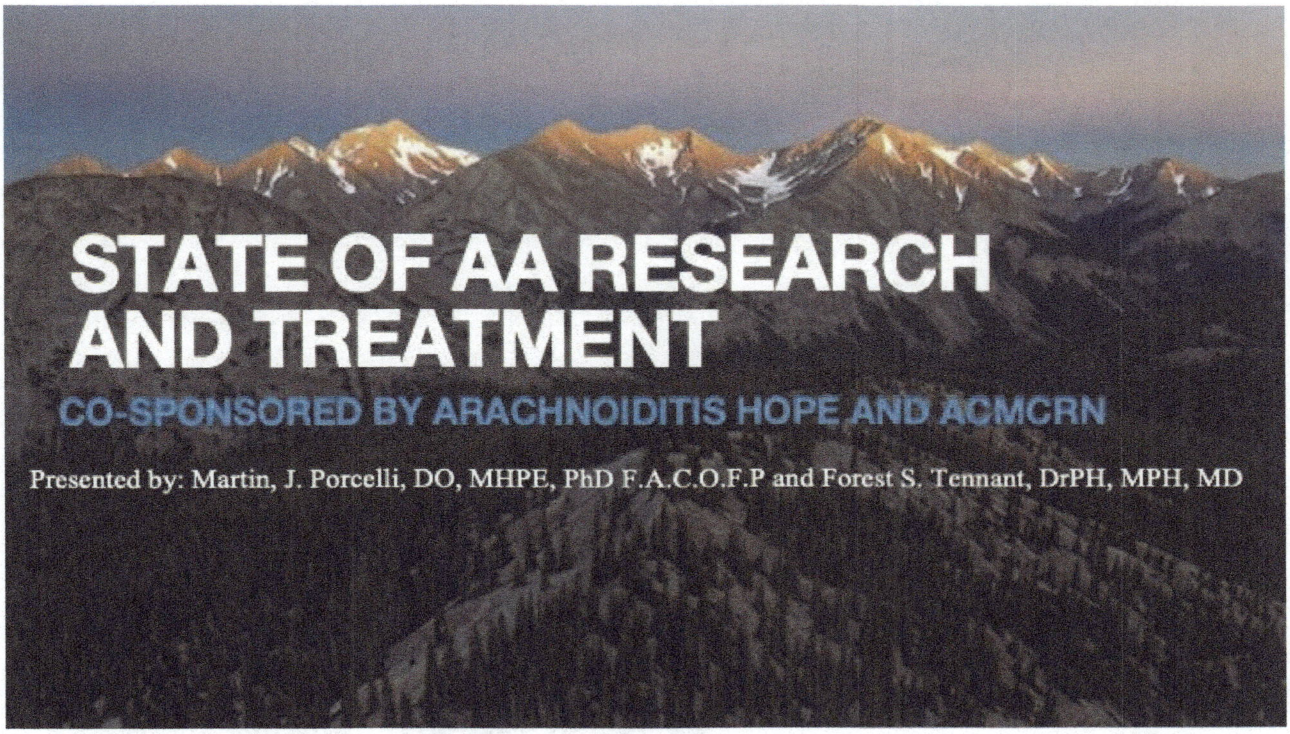

Presenter Disclosure:

The presenter, Dr. Porcelli, has no relevant financial relationships with commercial entities to disclose. This presentation does not involve the discussions of off-label or investigational uses of products or devices

Keywords:

- Adhesive Arachnoiditis
- Chronic Pain
- Autoimmune
- MRI
- Multidisciplinary Treatment
- Spinal Procedures
- Cytokines
- Medication

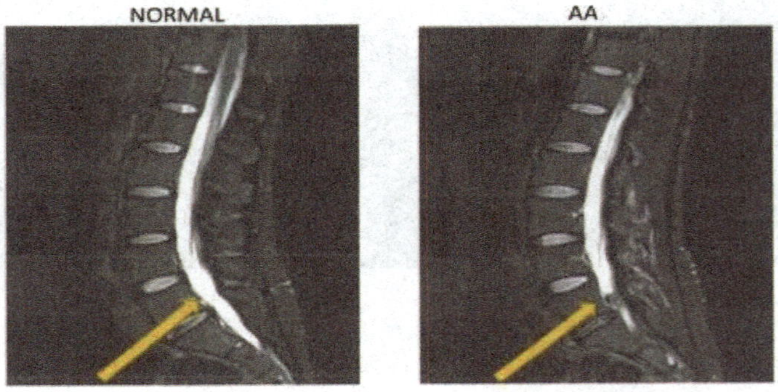

Normal lateral view of the spinal canal. The white is spinal fluid. Normally a gray color inside the spinal canal represents the spinal cord or the cauda equina nerve roots. A gray color may also indicate a disease process is present.

The arrow points to a clump of nerve roots that has resulted from inflammation and adhesions. There is adherence of the mass to the arachnoid-dural canal covering as well as spinal fluid flow obstruction.

Introduction to Arachnoiditis (ARC)

Definition & Historical Context

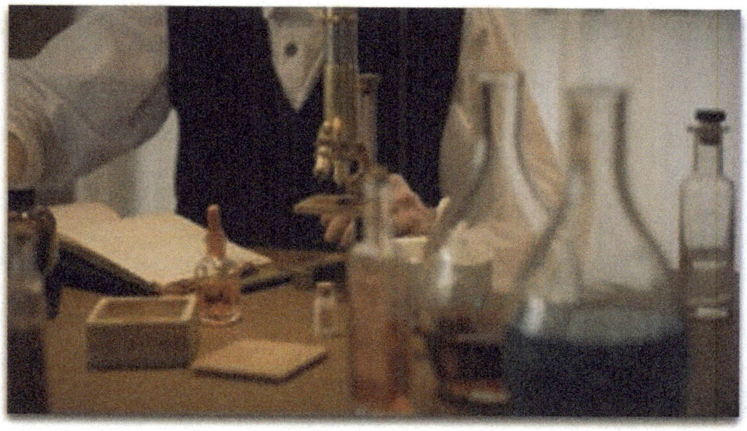

- First defined in **1872** as inflammation of the **arachnoid membrane,** the middle layer of the meninges.
- Known historically as the **"Devil's Disease"** due to severe pain, suffering, and high mortality.
- **Common early causes**: Tuberculosis and syphilis.
- Dr. Thomas Addison noted spinal pathology consistent with ARC in 1855 adrenal cases.
- **No effective treatment** existed in the 19th and 20th centuries; often seen as untreatable.

Emergence of Adhesive Arachnoiditis (AA)

Medical Discovery & Focus

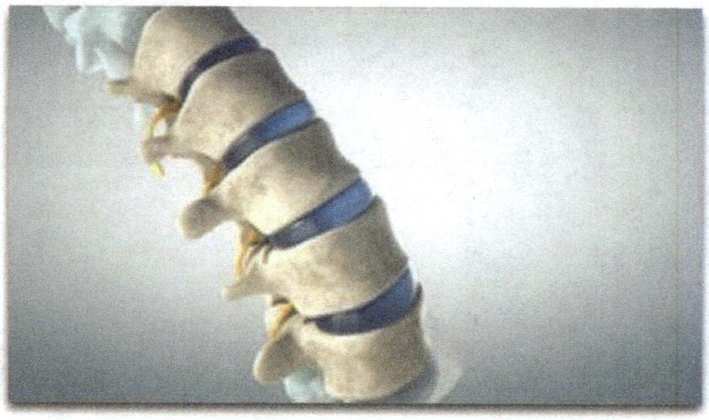

- In early 1900s, **Horsley and Harvey** identified **adhesions** gluing **cauda equina nerve roots** to the arachnoid membrane.
- Term **Adhesive Arachnoiditis (AA)** coined to describe this specific condition.
- **Focus today** is on **lumbar-sacral AA**, now more commonly diagnosed in clinical practice.
- This study reports preliminary diagnostic and clinical efforts targeting lumbar-sacral **AA**.

Epidemiology of AA

- **Difficult to quantify** due to varied symptoms and historical underdiagnosis
- **Improved imaging & awareness** have led to more identified cases
- Historically linked to **infections** and **medical procedures**; re-emerging with increased spinal interventions
- Though **not common,** AA has a **significant impact** on those affected
- **More research** is needed to understand its true prevalence and burden
- Over 50 foreign countries have submitted **MRI** evident to the foundation for further elaboration

Methods

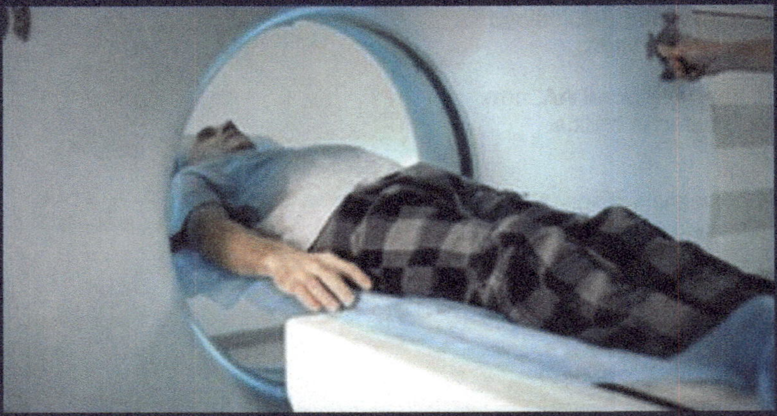

Project Overview

- **Tennant Foundation** – Adhesive Arachnoiditis Study & Education Project
- Created in response to the **severe nature of AA** and **limited clinical data**
- Goal: Collect **demographic and clinical data** to guide diagnosis and treatment
- Primary method: Review of **MRI-documented AA cases** and clinical info
- Approved by the Institutional Review Committee of the Tennant Foundation
- Case submissions accepted from **patients, families, and physicians**

Tennant Foundation

Case Collection & Global Reach

- MRI and case review requests shared via AA social media groups
- Cases received from **50+ countries**, indicating global recognition of AA
- All participants signed a release for de-identified educational use
- **No cost** or compensation involved for participants
- No medications prescribed or labs conducted during the study

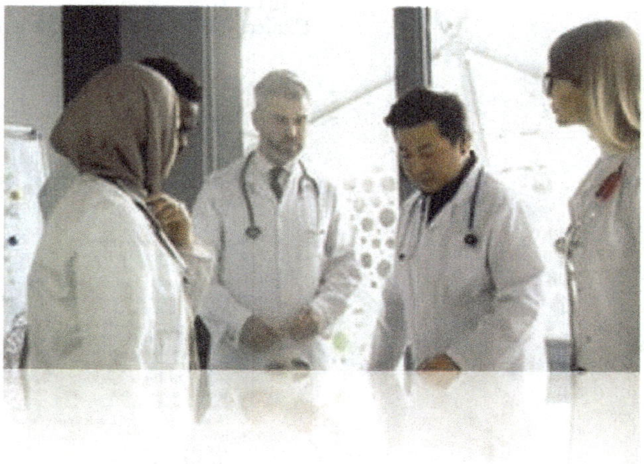

Data & Diagnostic Basis

- Initial analysis based on **80 consecutive AA cases**
- Focused diagnostic and treatment insights drawn from:
    - A. Published literature
    - B. Clinical and anecdotal observations
    - C. **80 MRI-confirmed AA cases** treated in a clinical practice
- Findings help guide future diagnostic and therapeutic strategies

Here are AXIAL (head-to-toe) VIEWS of the Lumbar-Sacral Canal at about L4 – 5:

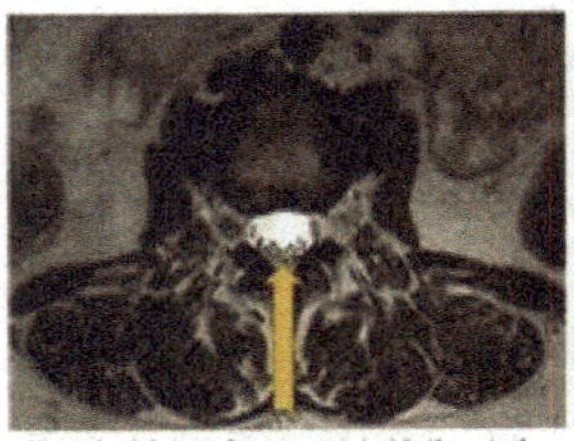

Normal axial view of nerve roots inside the spinal canal. The white is spinal fluid. Note size, placement, and symmetry of the nerve roots.

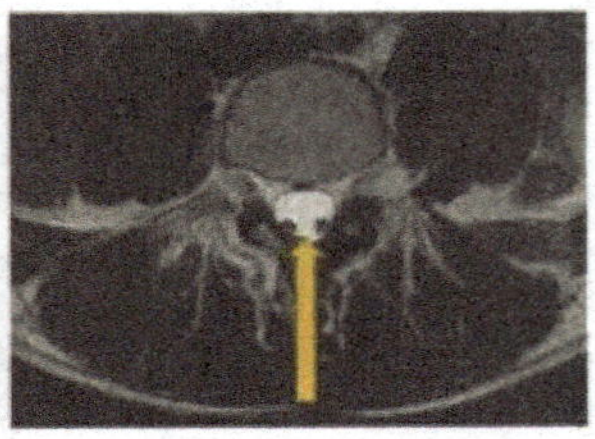

Adhesive arachnoiditis. Note the asymmetry, mass formation, and attachment of the nerve root clumps to the arachnoid-dural covering.

Data & Diagnostic Basis

TABLE 1:
Clinical Profile of 80 MRI-Documented Cases of AA

NO.	
1. Females	65 – 81%
2. Males	15 – 19%
3. Age Range in Years	18 to 80
4. Mean Age ± S.D. in Years	48.9 ± 13.7
5. No. with a Predisposing Spinal Condition'	61 – 76.3%
a. Herniated discs	44 – 55%
b. Spondylolisthesis	17 – 21.25%
c. Osteoporosis	6 – 7.5%
d. Spine arthritis	23 – 28.75%
e. Scoliosis	9 – 11.25%
f. Tarlov cysts	9 – 11.25%
6. No. with One or More Spinal Surgeries	43 – 53.8%
7. Total No. of Spine Surgeries in 43 Cases	91
8. Range of Surgeries in 43 Cases	1 to 8
9. No. Who Had two or More Spine Surgeries	22 – 27.5%
10. No. Who Had One or More Epidural Injections	69 – 86.3%
11. Total No. Epidural Injections in 69 Cases	236
12. Range of Epidural Injections in 69 Cases	1 to 20
13. No. Reported Over 8 Epidural Injections	16 – 20.0%
14. Symptoms and Complications Reported by Over 55% of Cases	
a. Pain Relief on standing	70 – 87.5%
b. Standing Too Long Causes Need to Lie Down	69 – 86.3%
c. Hurts to Lie Flat on Back	67 – 83.8%
d. Pain Always Present	66 – 82.5%
e. Shooting Pains, Tremors, or Jerking in Legs	64 – 78.8%
f. Burning Pains in Feet	63 – 78.8%
g. Cold Hands or Feet	58 – 72.5%
h. Crawling of Insects on Skin	58 – 72.5%
i. Water Dripping/Running Down Legs	53 – 66.3%
j. Difficulties Starting Urination/Defecation	51 – 63.8%
k. Leg Raise Hurts Back	50 – 62.5%
l. Blurred Vision	47 – 58.8%
m. Pain Behind Eyes	45 – 56.3%

Pathophysiology of AA

- **Rise in AA diagnoses** parallels the **increase in back pain** this century
  - Contributing factors: **Sedentary lifestyle, obesity, poor posture, diet, and seating ergonomics**
- **Advanced MRI technology has improved detection of AA**
- **Most common precursor: Herniated discs**
- **Key risk factors:**
  - **Genetic: Ehlers-Danlos Syndrome**
  - **Autoimmune: Lupus, rheumatoid spondylitis**
  - **Structural: Scoliosis, spondylolisthesis**
  - **Trauma & Medical procedures:** Especially **epidural injections & spinal surgeries**
- **AA is multifactorial, often developing after a combination of predisposing conditions and interventions**

Clinical Profile of AA

- **Typically presents as chronic back pain unresponsive to standard treatments**
- **Based on review of 80 MRI-documented cases (2022 Study)**

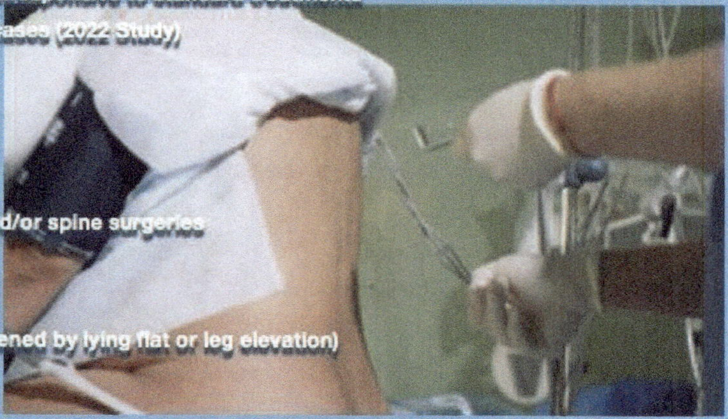

Common Patient Profile:

- **Middle-aged female**
- **History of spinal abnormalities**
- **Underwent multiple epidural injections and/or spine surgeries**

Major Symptoms:

- **Constant pain (relieved by standing, worsened by lying flat or leg elevation)**
- **Urinary difficulties**
- **Blurred vision**
- **Unusual sensations:**
  - **Feeling of insects crawling or water running down the legs**

Physical Examination

🔍 Key Observations:

- No *specific* physical signs confirm AA
- However, abnormal physical symptoms are usually present

Neurological & Musculoskeletal Findings:

- Lower extremity weakness
- Diminished reflexes
- Positive Straight Leg Raise
  - Pain elicited or motion restricted

Structural & Soft Tissue Changes:

- Muscle contraction & soft tissue indentations in the back
  - Caused by pain-induced splinting
  - May result from spinal fluid leakage

⚠ Spinal Fluid Toxicity:

- Spinal fluid is a **toxic irritant**
  - Irritates muscles and soft tissues
  - Leads to spinal muscle atrophy

TABLE 2.
Symptoms and Complications Reported by Over 55% of Cases

a. Pain relief on standing	70-87.5%
b. Standing too long Causes need to lie down	69-86.3%
c. Hurts to lie flat on back	67-83.8%
d. Pain always present	66-82.5%
e. Shooting pains, tremors, or jerking in the legs	64-78.8%
f. Burning pains/neuropathies in feet	63-78.8%
g. Cold hands or feet	58-72.5%
h. Crawling of insects on skin	58-72.5%
i. Water dripping/running down legs	53-66.3%
j. Difficulties starting urination/ defecation	51-63.8%
k. Leg raise hurts back	50-62.5%
l. Blurred vision	47-58.8%
m. Pain behind eyes (retrobulbar)	45-56.3%

Laboratory Testing

Key Concept:

- Arachnoiditis is an inflammatory disease
- Inflammatory markers are often **elevated in lab tests**

📊 Common Abnormal Laboratory Findings:

- Elevated White Blood Cell Count (WBC)
- Increased Erythrocyte Sedimentation Rate (ESR/SED Rate)
- Elevated C-Reactive Protein (CRP)
- Increased Cytokines & Interleukins
  - Especially with degenerative disc disease (DDD)

📌 Clinical Insight:

- Degenerated intervertebral discs may trigger cytokine elevation
- These findings are **typical in AA patients**

Imaging Follow-up:

- MRI is required to confirm AA
- **Abnormal labs** may indicate the **need for MRI**

TABLE 1:
Clinical Profile of 80 MRI-Documented Cases of AA

NO.	
1. Females	65 – 81%
2. Males	15 – 19%
3. Age Range in Years	18 to 80
4. Mean Age ± S.D. in Years	48.9 ± 13.7
5. No. with a Predisposing Spinal Condition*	61 – 76.3%
a. Herniated discs	44 – 55%
b. Spondylolisthesis	17 – 21.25%
c. Osteoporosis	6 – 7.5%
d. Spine arthritis	23 – 28.75%
e. Scoliosis	9 - 11.25%
f. Tarlov cysts	9 - 11.25%
6. No. with One or More Spinal Surgeries	43 – 53.8%
7. Total No. of Spine Surgeries in 43 Cases	91
8. Range of Surgeries in 43 Cases	1 to 8
9. No. Who Had two or More Spine Surgeries	22 – 27.5%
10. No. Who Had One or More Epidural Injections	69 – 86.3%
11. Total No. Epidural Injections in 69 Cases	236
12. Range of Epidural Injections in 69 Cases	1 to 20
13. No. Reported Over 8 Epidural Injections	16 – 20.0%
14. Symptoms and Complications Reported by Over 55% of Cases	
a. Pain Relief on standing	70 – 87.5%
b. Standing Too Long Causes Need to Lie Down	69 – 86.3%
c. Hurts to Lie Flat on Back	67 – 83.8%
d. Pain Always Present	66 – 82.5%
e. Shooting Pains, Tremors, or Jerking in Legs	64 – 78.8%
f. Burning Pains in Feet	63 – 78.8%
g. Cold Hands or Feet	58 – 72.5%
h. Crawling of Insects on Skin	58 – 72.5%
i. Water Dripping/Running Down Legs	53 – 66.3%
j. Difficulties Starting Urination/Defecation	51 – 63.8%
k. Leg Raise Hurts Back	50 – 62.5%
l. Blurred Vision	47 – 58.8%
m. Pain Behind Eyes	45 – 56.3%

Staging and Classification

Stage One – Mild

- Extremities: full range of motion, strength, extension
- No urinary or central symptoms*
- Normal ambulation
- Low-level pain: non-opioid management is sufficient

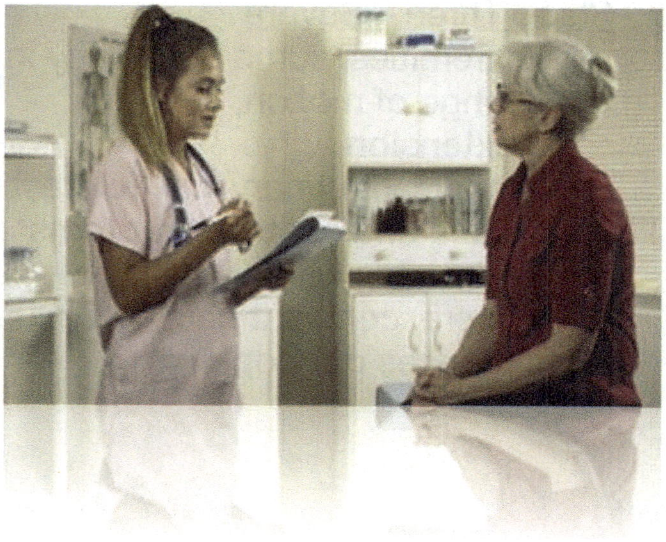

Staging and Classification (cont.)

Stage Two – Moderate

- Extremities: full range of motion, strength, extension
- Some urinary, gastrointestinal tract, and central symptoms*
- Normal ambulation
- Constant pain: non-opioid management is sufficient

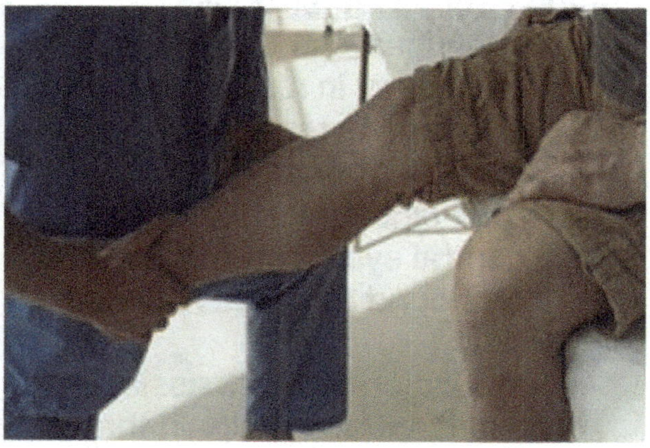

Staging and Classification (cont.)

<u>Stage Three – Severe</u>

- Extremities: some deficiency in range of motion, strength, extension
- Significant urinary, gastrointestinal tract, and central symptoms*
- Ambulates with assistance+
- Severe, constant pain that usually requires daily opioids

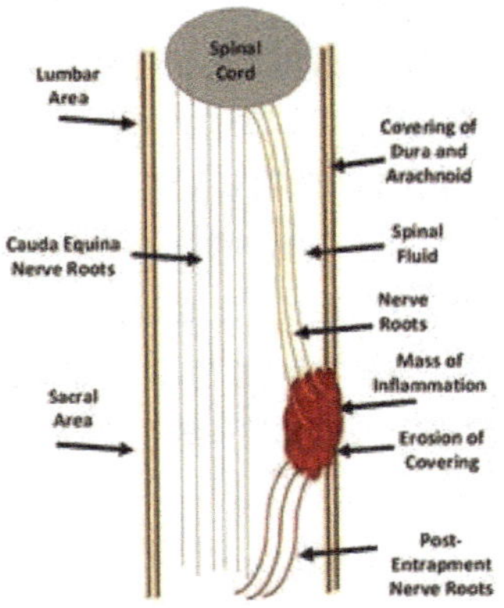

Staging and Classification (cont.)

<u>Stage Four – Catastrophic</u>

- Extremities: significant deficiency in range of motion, strength, extension
- Significant urinary, gastrointestinal tract, and central symptoms*
- Bed bound all or part of each day
- Ambulation requires assistance
- Severe, intractable pain that requires palliative care

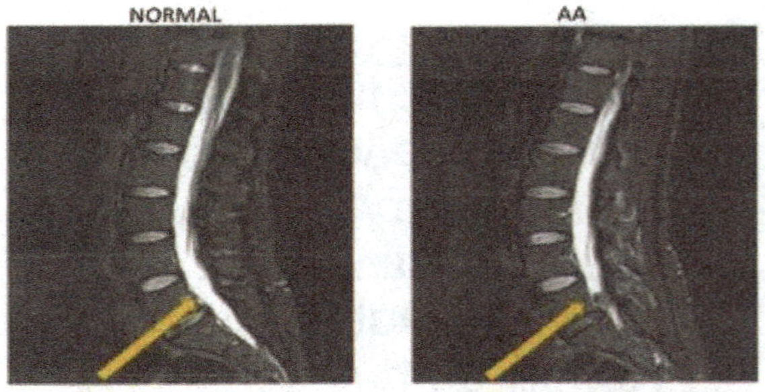

Normal lateral view of the spinal canal. The white is spinal fluid. Normally a gray color inside the spinal canal represents the spinal cord or the cauda equina nerve roots. A gray color may also indicate a disease process is present.

The arrow points to a clump of nerve roots that has resulted from inflammation and adhesions. There is adherence of the mass to the arachnoid-dural canal covering as well as spinal fluid flow obstruction.

Complications	Consequences
SPINAL FLUID FLOW OBSTRUCTION	➢ Headache ➢ Blurred vision ➢ Tinnitus (Ringing in ears) ➢ Mental impairments (memory, attention, reading, and mathematical ability)
SPINAL FLUID FLOW LEAKAGE	➢ Contraction of paraspinal muscles ➢ Tissue over lumbar spine indents or "caves in" ➢ Arms can't extend
SITTING/STANDING ABILITY IMPAIRED	➢ Can't sit or stand in one position very long
INTRACTABLE PAIN SYNDROME	➢ Constant ("24/7") pain ➢ Cardiovascular, metabolic, and endocrine dysfunctions

Complications	Consequences
NEUROPATHIC SYMPTOMS	➢ Burning feet ➢ Shooting pains into buttocks or legs ➢ Radiating type pain
IMPAIRED IMMUNITY	➢ Sepsis (infection) ➢ Premature death
LOSS OF BLADDER, BOWEL, AND SEXUAL FUNCTION	➢ Urgency, incontinence, hesitancy, or paralysis ➢ Bloating, abdominal pain, alternating constipation, and diarrhea ➢ Sex organs disabled, loss of libido
LEG AND FOOT PARALYSIS	➢ Weakness ➢ Inability to stand or walk ➢ Foot drop

Complications	Consequences
BIZARRE NEUROLOGIC SYMPTOMS	➢ Sensation of water or insects on legs ➢ Burning of feet or buttocks ➢ Leg jerking, spasms, "restless legs"
DIETARY DYSFUNCTION	➢ Loss of appetite ➢ Excess sugar intake ➢ Malnutrition/weight loss ➢ Anorexia
HORMONAL DEFICIENCIES	➢ Cortisol ➢ Pregnenolone ➢ Dehydroepiandrosterone (DHEA) ➢ Testosterone

Treatments

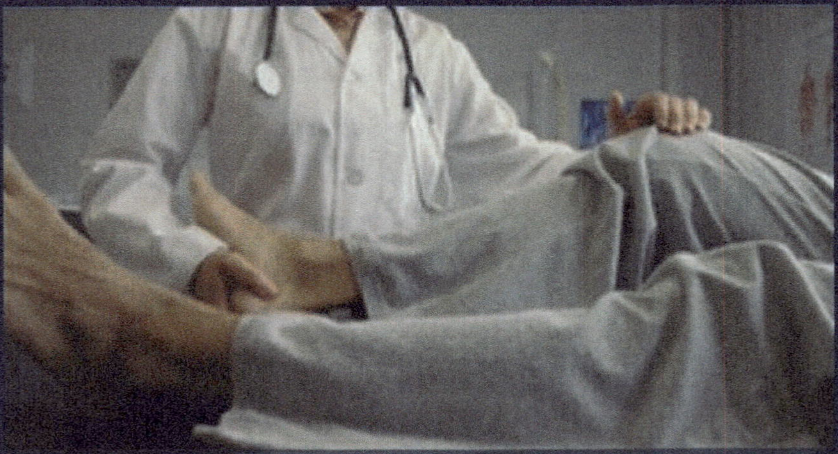

A New Approach to AA Treatment

- **Past belief**: "Nothing can be done" — now **outdated**
- **Today**: Positive outcomes reported in the Study & Education Project
  - Pain relief
  - Improved physical & mental function
  - Slowed or halted disease progression

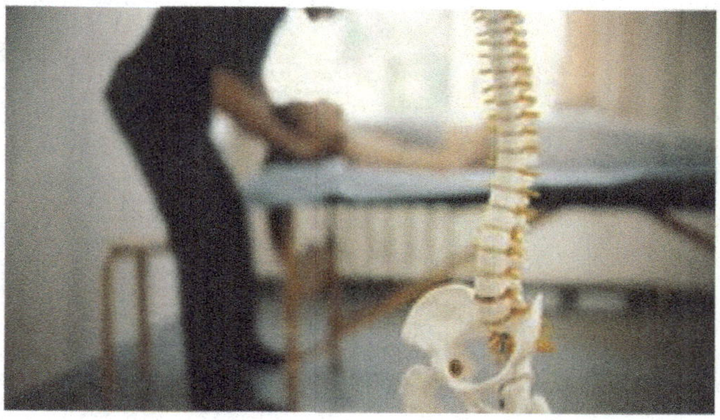

Three-Part Treatment Strategy:

1. Neuroinflammation suppression
2. Neuroregeneration
3. Pain control

Pharmacologic & Anti-Inflammatory Measures

Key Treatments:

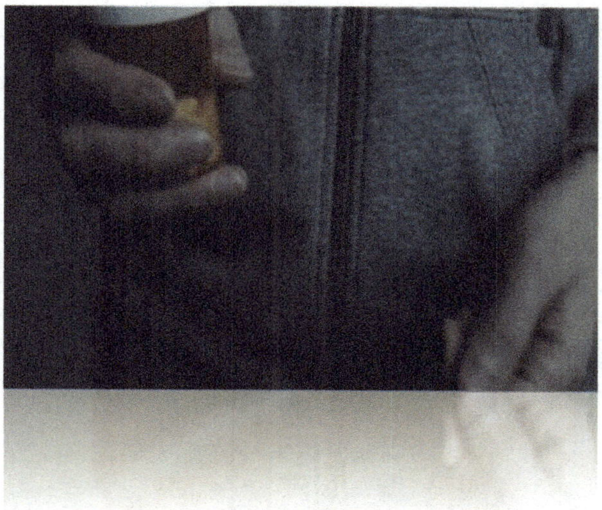

- Low-Dose Naltrexone (LDN)
  - Start: 1–7 mg 1–2x/day, titrate up to max 14 mg/day
  - Helps both pain relief and inflammation suppression
- Intermittent anti-inflammatories (1–3x/week):
  - Ketorolac (10–30 mg)
  - Methylprednisolone (2–4 mg)
  - Dexamethasone (.5–.75 mg)
  - **Other NSAIDs:** Diclofenac, meloxicam, indomethacin

Pain Relief

While Staying Under 90MME

MAXIMAL DAILY OPIOID DOSAGES
FOR 90 MG MORPHINE EQUIVALENCE

MAXIMAL DAILY OPIOID DOSAGES ALLOWED	
Approx. Oral Doses a Day	OPIOID (Oral or Patch)
8-9	Morphine – 10 mg
3-4	Methadone – 10 mg
8-9	Hydrocodone/APAP – 10/325 mg (Vicodin®, Norco®)
3	Morphine – 30 mg
6	Oxycodone/APAP – 10/325 mg (Percocet®)
5	Hydromorphone – 4 mg (Dilaudid®)
2-3	Hydromorphone – 8 mg (Dilaudid®)
6	Oxycodone Plain – 10 mg
2-3	Oxycodone Plain – 20 mg
2	Oxycodone Plain – 30 mg
16-20	Codeine 30 mg
8-10	Codeine 60 mg
16-18	Tramadol 50 mg
8-9	Tramadol 100 mg
1	Fentanyl Patch – 25 mcg per hour
1	Fentanyl Patch – 50 mcg per hour is 120 mg of morphine equivalence
	OPIOID INJECTIONS
2-4	Hydromorphone 50 mg/ml, .05 to .1 ml (2.5 to 5 mg)
3-4	Fentanyl 1000 mcg/ml, 0.1 ml (100 mcg) sub cu per injection
8-9	Morphine 10 mg per injection
3-4	Meperidine (Demerol®) 50-100 mg per injection
• This table is based on recommendations of the Federal Centers for Medicare and Medicaid.	
• If a patient wishes, they can take 2 opioids, each at half the maximal number a day which is listed above.	

Pain Relief

While Staying Under 90MME

- Descending pain
- Injectable hydromorphone
- Ketorolac
- Gabapentin
- Medrol
- Diomax
- Policy

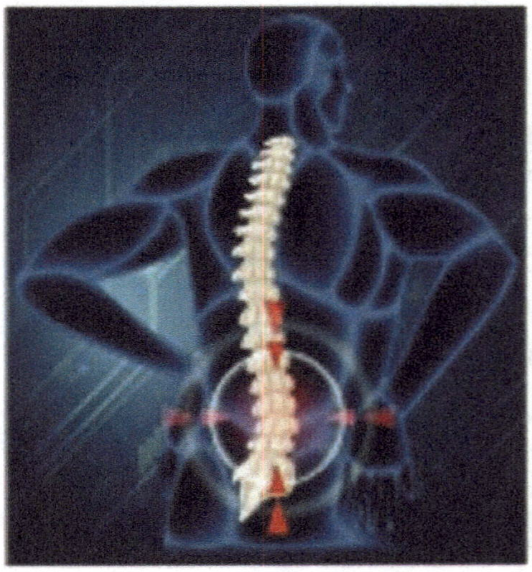

Conclusion: Renewed Understanding of Adhesive Arachnoiditis (AA)

- Resurgence of AA linked to advanced MRI diagnostics, improving detection
- Common in patients with chronic back pain unresponsive to standard treatments
- Symptoms: Urinary dysfunction, neurological sensations
- Causes:
  - Disc degeneration
  - Genetic & autoimmune factors
  - Post-surgical or procedural trauma

Current Treatments (though not from clinical trials):

- Inflammation suppression
- Neuroregeneration strategies
- Pain management
- Physical medicine remains valuable

- Call to Action:
  - Medical community must stay vigilant and proactive
  - Urgent need to refine diagnostics and develop new therapies

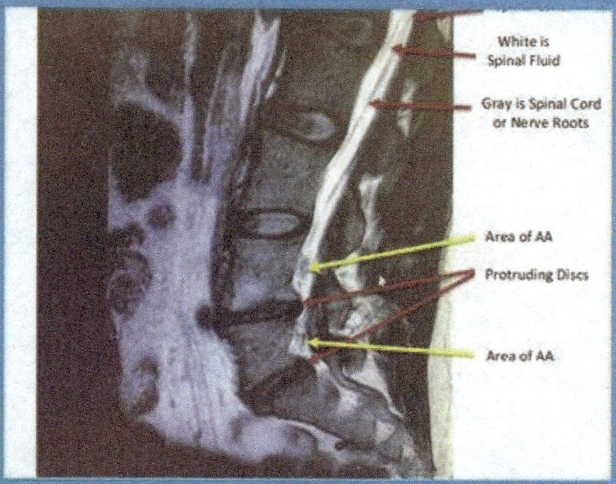

Neuroregeneration & Physical Therapies

Neuroregeneration Support:

- Hormones & polypeptides:
  - **DHEA (dehydroepiandrosterone), colostrum, nandrolone** (for nutritional deficiencies)
- High-protein diet with collagen/amino acid supplements
- Check for nutritional deficiencies

Physical Measures:

- Daily leg and foot exercises
  - Stretching, straight-leg raises, foot flexing, walking
- Flexibility & mobility therapies
  - OMT (Osteopathic Manipulative Treatment), stretching, slow movement
- Ancillary therapies:
  - Water soaking
  - Electromedical therapy

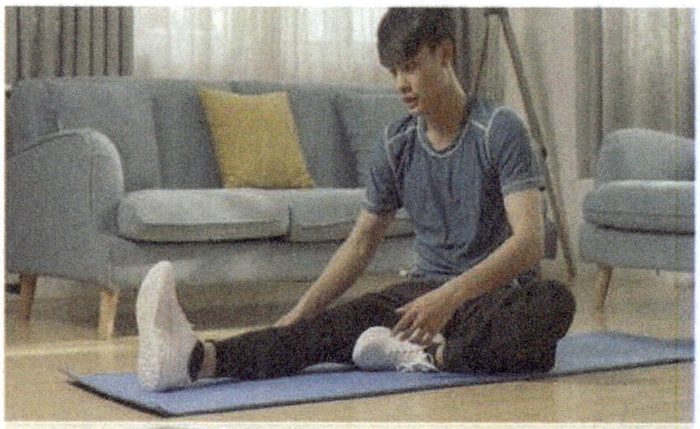

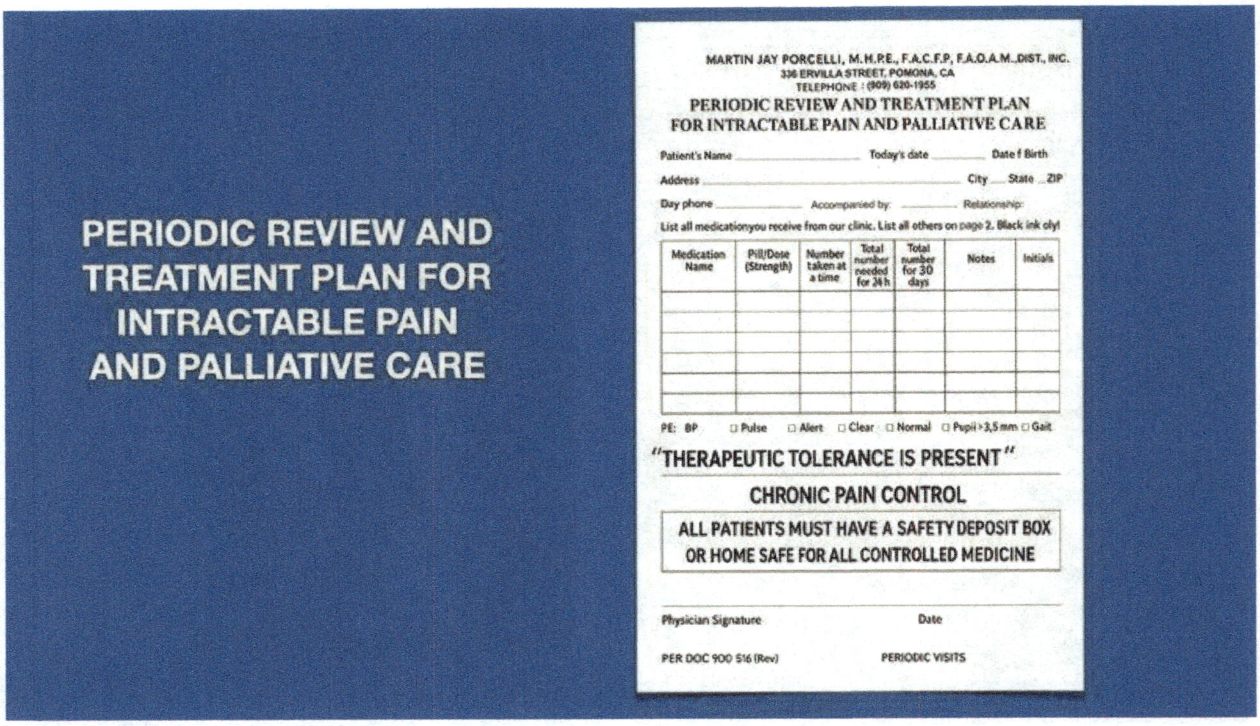
PERIODIC REVIEW AND TREATMENT PLAN FOR INTRACTABLE PAIN AND PALLIATIVE CARE
MARTIN JAY PORCELLI, M.H.P.E., F.A.C.F.P, F.A.O.A.M..DIST., INC.
336 ERVILLA STREET, POMONA, CA
TELEPHONE : (909) 620-1955
PERIODIC REVIEW AND TREATMENT PLAN FOR INTRACTABLE PAIN AND PALLIATIVE CARE
Patient's Name
Today's date
Date f Birth
Address
City
State
ZIP
Day phone
Accompanied by:
Relationship:
List all medicationyou receive from our clinic. List all others on page 2. Black ink oly!
Medication Name
Pill/Dose (Strength)
Number taken at a time
Total number needed for 24 h
Total number for 30 days
Notes
Initials
PE: BP
□ Pulse
□ Alert
□ Clear
□ Normal
□ Pupil >3,5 mm
□ Gait
"THERAPEUTIC TOLERANCE IS PRESENT"
CHRONIC PAIN CONTROL
ALL PATIENTS MUST HAVE A SAFETY DEPOSIT BOX OR HOME SAFE FOR ALL CONTROLLED MEDICINE
Physician Signature
Date
PER DOC 900 516 (Rev)
PERIODIC VISITS

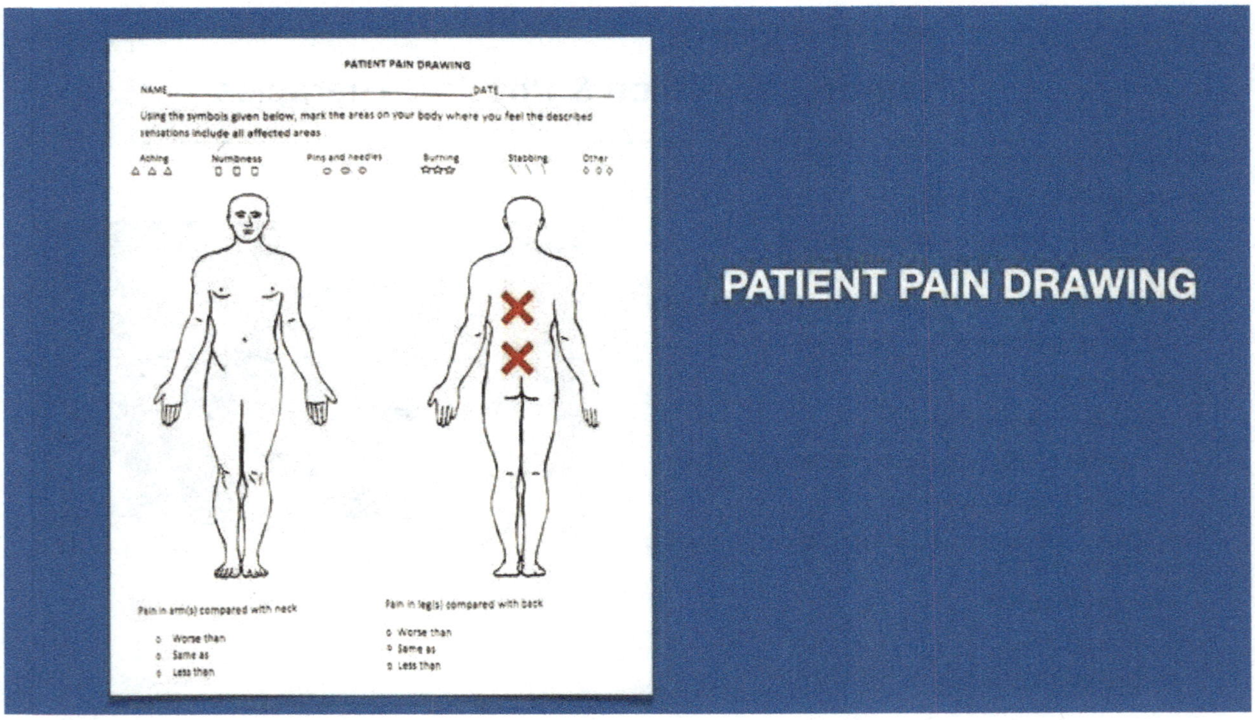
PATIENT PAIN DRAWING
NAME
DATE
Using the symbols given below, mark the areas on your body where you feel the described sensations include all affected areas
Aching
Numbness
Pins and needles
Burning
Stabbing
Other
Pain in arm(s) compared with neck
Worse than
Same as
Less than
Pain in leg(s) compared with back
Worse than
Same as
Less than
PATIENT PAIN DRAWING

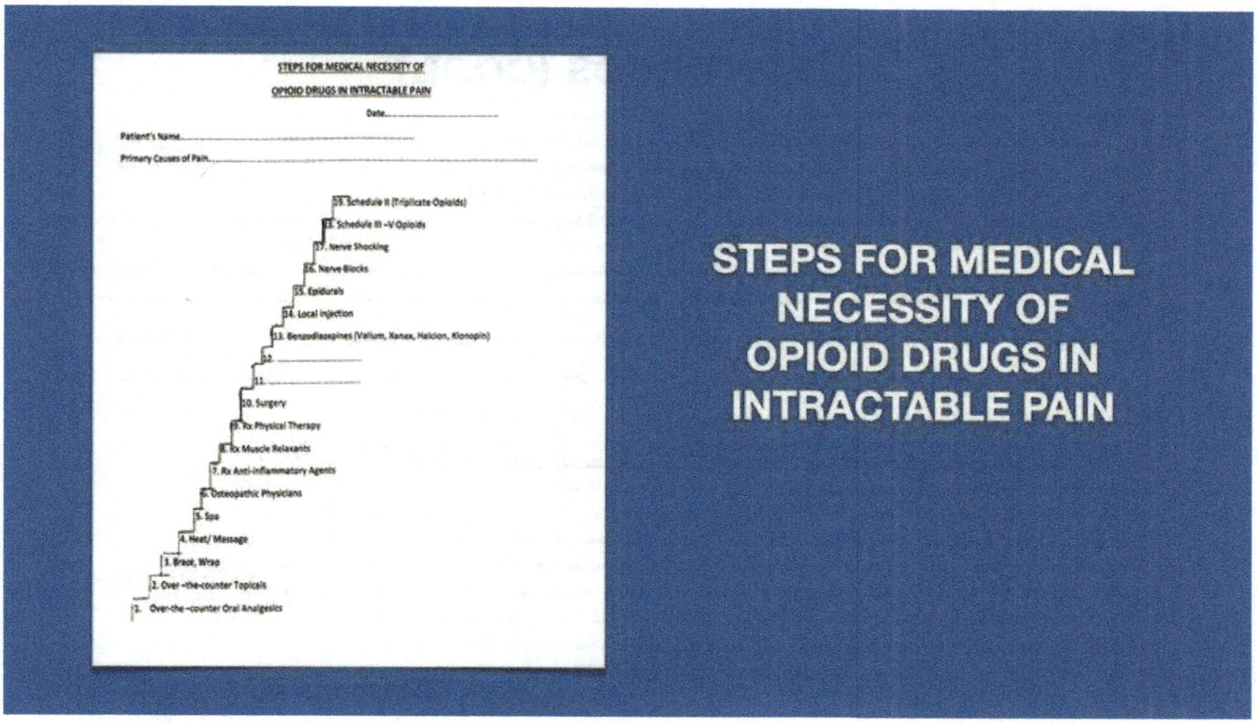

References

1. Thomas J. Arachnitis and Arachnoiditis. In: Comprehensive Medical Dictionary. Philadelphia, PA: J.B. Lippincott & Co; 1873:57.
2. Damkier HH, Brown PD, Praetorius J. Cerebrospinal fluid secretion by the choroid plexus. Physiol Rev. 2013;93(4):1847-1892.
3. Kiski H, Aanismaa R, Tenhunen J, et al. Healthy human CSF promotes glial differentiation of hESC-derived neural cells while retaining spontaneous activity in existing neuronal networks. Biol Open. 2013;2(6):605-612.
4. Aldrete JA. History and evaluation of arachnoiditis: The evidence revealed. Insurgentes Centro 51-A. Col San Rafael, Mexico. 2010:3-14.
5. Aldrete JA. Arachnoiditis: The Silent Epidemic. Mexico: Future Med Publishers; 2003.
6. Addison T. On the Constitutional and Local Effects of Disease of the Supra-Renal Capsules. London, England: Samuel Highley; 1855.
7. Harvey SC. Meningeal adhesions and their significance. Interstate Post Grad Med. 1926;2:27-31.
8. Horsley V. Chronic spinal meningitis: it's differential diagnosis and surgical treatment. Br J Med. 1909;1:513-517.
9. Maillard J, Batista S, Medeiros F, et al. Spinal Adhesive Arachnoiditis: A Literature Review. Cureus. 2023;15(1):e33697. Published 2023 Jan 12. doi:10.7759/cureus.33697
10. Quiles M, Marchisello PJ, Tsairis P. Lumbar adhesive arachnoiditis: Etiologic and pathologic aspects. Spine. 1978;3(1):45-50.
11. Todeschi J, Chibbaro S, Gubian A, Pop R, Proust F, Cebula H. Spinal adhesive arachnoiditis following the rupture of an Adamkiewicz aneurysm: Literature review and a case illustration. Neurochirurgie. 2018 Jun;64(3):177-182.
12. Ross JS, Masaryk TS, Modic MT, et al. MRI imaging of lumbar arachnoiditis. AJR Am J Roentgenol. 1987;149(5):1025-1032.
13. Bourne IH. Lumbosacral adhesive arachnoiditis: A review. J R Soc Med. 1990;83(4):262-265.
14. Delamarter RB, Ross JS, Masaryk TS, et al. Diagnosis of lumbar arachnoiditis by magnetic resonance imaging. Spine. 1990;15(3):304-310.
15. Shiraishi T, Crook HV, Reynolds A. Spinal arachnoiditis ossificans: Observations on its investigation and treatment. Eur Spine J. 1995;4(1):60-63.
16. Stookey B. Adhesive spinal arachnoiditis simulating spinal cord tumor. Arch Neurol Psychiatry. 1927;17:151-164.
17. Dahlhamer J, Lucas J, Zelaya C, et al. Prevalence of chronic and high-impact chronic pain among adults, United States, 2016. MMWR Morb Mortal Wkly Rep. 2018 Sep 14;67(36):1001-1006.
18. Hoy D, March L, Brooks P, et al. The global burden of low back pain: estimates from the Global Burden of Disease 2010 study. Ann Rheum Dis. 2014;73(6):968-974.
19. Smith M, Davis MA, Stano M, et al. Aging baby boomers and the rising cost of chronic back pain: secular trend analysis of longitudinal medical expenditures panel survey data from 2000 to 2007. J Manipulative Physiol Ther. 2013;36(1):2-11.
20. Strine TW, Hootman JM. US national prevalence and correlation of low back and neck pain among adults. Arthritis Rheum. 2007;57(3):656-665.

References (cont.)

21.Andersson GB. Epidemiological features of chronic low back pain. Lancet. 1999;354(9178):582-585.

22.Deyo RA, Dvorkin SF, Antmann D, et al. Report of the NIH Task Force on chronic low back pain research standards. J Pain. 2014;115(2):569-585.

23.Deyo RA, Mirza SK, Martin BI. Back pain prevalence and visit rates: estimates from U.S. national surveys, 2002. Spine. 2006;31(23):2724-2727.

24.Freburger JK, Holmes GM, Agans RP, et al. The rising prevalence of chronic low back pain. Arch Intern Med. 2009;169(3):251-258.

25.Jackson A, Isherwood I. Does degenerative disease of the lumbar spine cause arachnoiditis? A magnetic resonance study and review of the literature. Br J Radiol. 1994;67(797):840-847.

26.Jorgenson J, Hansen PH, Steenskoo V, et al. A clinical and radiological study of chronic lower spinal arachnoiditis. Neuroradiology. 1975;9(3):139-144.

27.Epstein NE. The risks of epidural and transforaminal steroid injections in the spine: commentary and a comprehensive review of the literature. Surg Neurol Int. 2013;4(Suppl 2):S574-S593.

28.Eisenberg E, Goldman R, Schlag-Eisenberg D, et al. Adhesive arachnoiditis following lumbar epidural steroid injections: A report of two cases and literature review. J Pain Res. 2019;12:513-518.

29.Todeschi J, Chibbaro S, Gubian A, Pop R, Proust F, Cebula H. Spinal adhesive arachnoiditis following the rupture of an Adamkiewicz aneurysm: Literature review and a case illustration. Neurochirurgie. 2018 Jun;64(3):177-182.

30.Anderson TL, Morris JM, Wald JT, Kotsenas AL. Imaging Appearance of Advanced Chronic Adhesive Arachnoiditis: A Retrospective Review. AJR Am J Roentgenol. 2017 Sep;209(3):648-655

31.Whedon JM, Glassey D. Cerebrospinal fluid stasis and its clinical significance. Altern Ther Health Med. 2009;15(2):54-60.

32.Tennant F. Adhesive Arachnoiditis: Identification, Treatment, and Management of Inflammatory Pain. Podiatry.com. Accessed January 11, 2024. https://www.podiatry.com/news/459/Adhesive-Arachnoiditis-Identification-Treatment-and-Management-of-Inflammatory-Pain

33.Arachnoiditis Hope website. https://arachnoiditishope.com/diagnosis/. Accessed January 19, 2024.

34.Parenti V, Huda F, Richardson PK, et al. Lumbar arachnoiditis: Does imaging associate with clinical features? Clin Neurol Neurosurg. 2020;192:105717.

35.Rodriguez LJG, Sandoval Sanchez V, Benavides Rodriguez D, et al. Paraplegia due to adhesive arachnoiditis: a case report. Acta Ortop Mex. 2009;23(4):232-236.

36.Bilello J, Tennant F. Patterns of chronic inflammation in extensively treated patients with arachnoiditis and chronic intractable pain. Postgrad Med. 2016;92(1096):1-5.

37.Zang Y, Chee A, Shi P, et al. Intervertebral disc cells produce interleukins found in patients with back pain. Am J Phys Med Rehabil. 2016;95(5):407-415.

38.Burns, L. Effects of Lumbar Lesions. The Educational Department A.T. Still Research Institute; Sunnyslope Laboratories; Academy of Applied Osteopathy.1966:62-63.

39.Arachnoiditis Hope website. https://arachnoiditishope.com/2020-aa-update-report/. Accessed January 19, 2024.

40.Arachnoiditis Hope website. https://arachnoiditishope.com/history/. Accessed January 19, 2024.

Acknowledgments

Thank you to Turquoise Video Productions, LLC for designing this presentation

Palliative Care for Advanced AA:Dr. Scott Guess

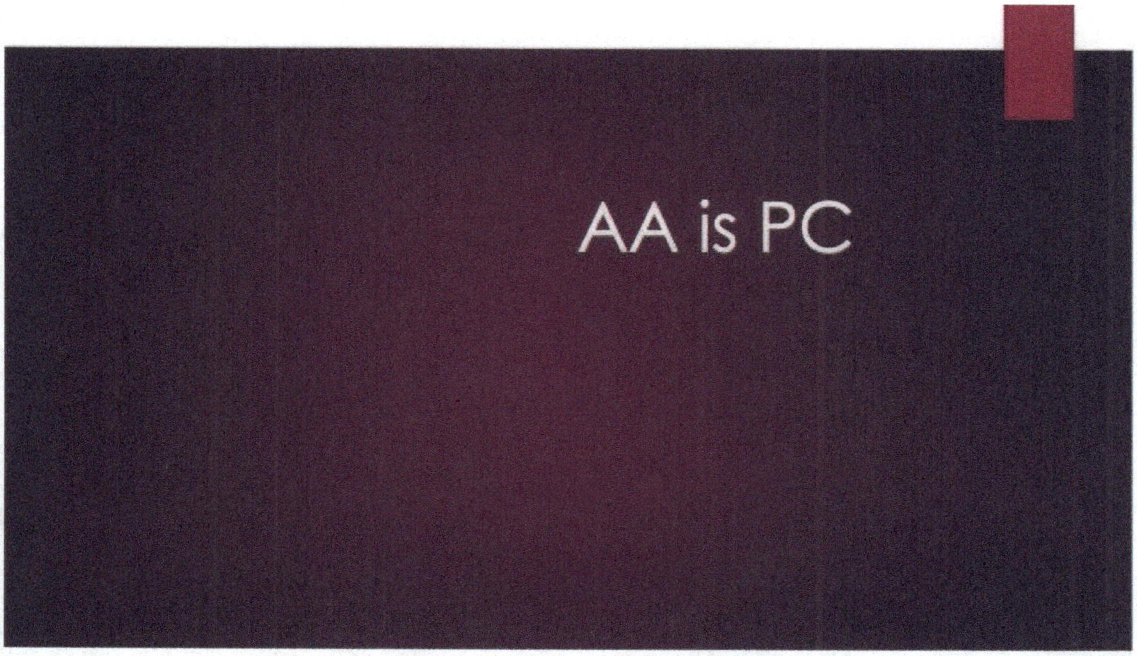

THERE IS NOTHING POLITICALLY CORRECT ABOUT ADHESIVE ARACHNOIDITIS

K. Scott Guess

- Doctor of Pharmacy
- Masters of Science Pharmaceutical Outcomes Process
- Masters of Science Palliative Care
- Registered Pharmacist
- Advanced Practice Pharmacist
- NO DISCLOSEURES

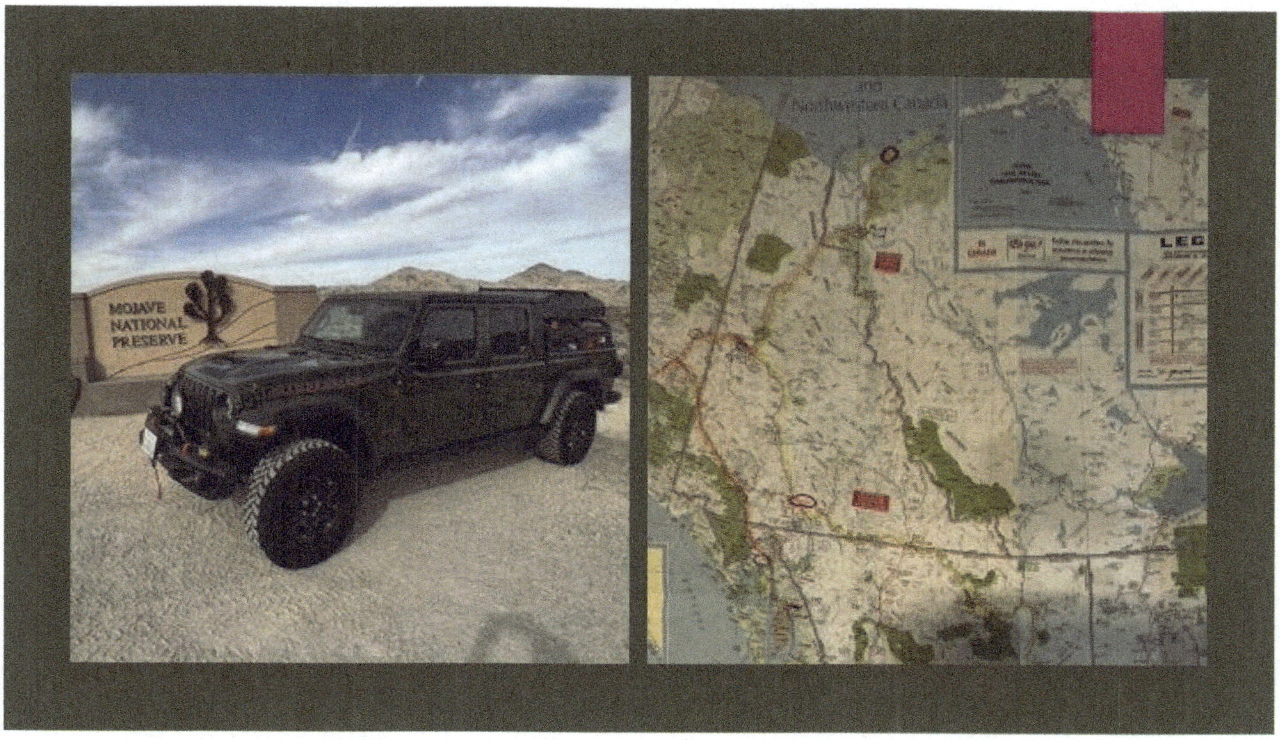

BY THE END OF THIS SESSION
I HOPE TO CONVINCE YOU
THAT
ADHESIVE ARACHNOIDITIS
IS A
PALLIATIVE CARE CONDITION

THE DIFFERENT CARE MODELS

PREVENTNIVE CARE

CURATIVE CARE

PALLIATIVE CARE

PREVENTITIVE CARE

AN OUCE OF PREVENTION IS WORTH A POUND OF CURE

MEDICAL INTERVENTIONS	LIFESTYLE PRACTICES	ANY PRECAUTION TO PREVENT ACCITENTAL INJURY
• VACCINATIONS • HEALTH SCREENINGS • DENTAL CARE AND CLEANINGS • MENTAL HEALTH SCREENINGS	• KEEPING THE BODY AND HEART STRONG THROUGH EXERCISE • EATING A HEALTHY DIET • MANAGING STRESS • Not Smoking/Quitting Smoking	

Center of Adult medicine and preventive care https://campmedicine.org/blog/examples-of-preventive-medicine-treatments-from-a-primary-physician
Kisling LA. Das JM. Prevention Strategies. [Updated 2023 Aug 1]. In: StatPearls [Internet]. Treasure Island (FL): StatPearls Publishing; 2023 Jan-. Available from: [illegible]
Types of preventive care. Rasmussen University. https://www.rasmussen.edu/degrees/health-sciences/blog/types-of-preventive-care

Curative Care

The stuff we can fix/cure

General Practice Care

- We can cure that infection
- We can cure some cancers now

Acute/Emergency/ Trauma Care

- We can set the broken bone
- We can sew up the cut
- We can dissolve that clot that caused the stroke or heart attack
- "We can rebuild him. We have the technology." (The Six Million Dollar Man)

Surgical Care

- We can resolve that appendicitis
- Gallstones/Kidney Stones
- Open Heart Surgery
- Organ transplants
- Hip/Knee/Shoulder replacements

Palliative Care

WHO Definition of Palliative Care

- **"Palliative care is an approach that improves the quality of life of patients and their families facing the problems associated with life-threatening illness, through the prevention and relief of suffering by means of early identification and impeccable assessments and treatment of pain and other problems, physical, psychosocial and spiritual (WHO 2002, p 83)"**

PALLIATIVE CARE IS FOR ALL THE STUFF WE CAN NOT FIX

THE STUFF WE JUST MANAGE – PALLIATE

The goal of palliative care is to diminish suffering and improve quality of life. Physical, Mental, Social and Spiritual suffering

Palliative Care Agenda

- **Pain control**
- Other symptom relief
  - Nause
  - Muscle spasm
  - Constipation
  - Anxiety
  - Depression
- Spiritual health
- Social heath
- Family health

Let me dispel a common misconception

PALLIATIVE CARE
IS NOT
HOSPICE CARE

Hospice is

- A FEDERAL BENEFIT PAID BY HHS THROUGH CMS
- IS INTENDED TO PROVIDE CARE DURING THE LAST 6 MONTHS OF LIFE

Hospice and palliative care share many of the same goals and principles with one notable exception

Palliative Care begins at the time the diagnosis

and

Lasts a lifetime

What kinds of conditions can you list that might be considered a palliative care diagnosis?

- Chronic anything
  - Pain
  - Cough
  - Headache
- Diabetes
- High blood pressure
- Congestive Heart Failure
- Alzheimer's/Dementia
- Cancers
- Organ diseases/failures
- Long Covid
- Congenital conditions
  - Multiple Sclerosis
  - Ehlers Danlos
  - Sickle Cell
- Structural Anomalies
  - Scoliosis
  - Chiari Malformations/Tarlov Cysts
  - Adhesive Arachnoiditis

Adhesive Arachnoiditis is

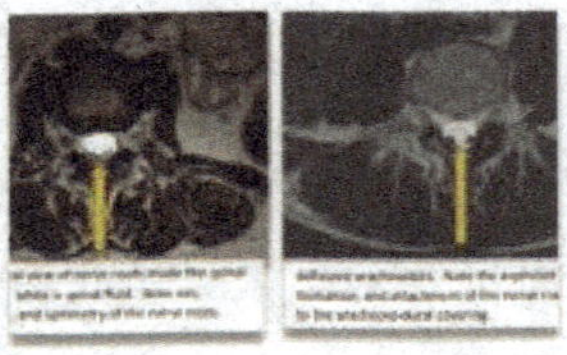

Most commonly the end of the spinal cord, the cauda equina,

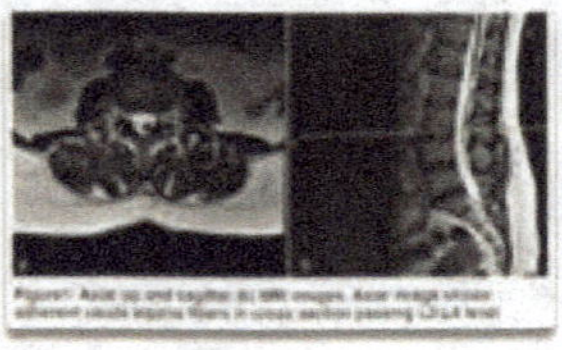

Clumped together by inflammation and

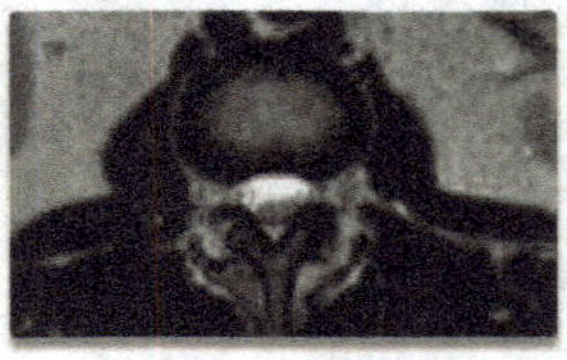

Trapped onto the wall of the spinal column, the arachnoid lining in scar tissue.

There is no cure

- We can not dissolve scar tissue anywhere
- We can surgically dissect out scar tissue in some locations like joints
- We can **not** remove scar tissue around nerves—especially within the spinal column

What we can do is…

- Reduce inflammation with
  - NSAID's but drug selection is critical here. As with all drug therapy for AA the drug MUST be able to pass through the blood brain barrier (BBB).

    NSAIDs Inhibit prostaglandins which start the pain and inflammatory process
    - Diclofenac (up to 100mg twice a day)
    - Ibuprofen (up to 800mg 4 times a day)
    - Flurbiprofen. (up to 100mg 3 times a day)
    - Indomethacin. (up do 50mg 4 times a day, ER 75mg 2 times a day)
  - Corticosteroids. – Reduces pro-inflammatory cytokines IL-6
    - Dexamethasone (1-4 mg daily, Dr. Tennant likes 3 times a week in the afternoon)
    - Methylprednisolone (4 mg daily, Dr. Tennant likes 3 times a week in the afternoon)
    - Prednisone/prednisolone. (1-5mg daily)

And this…

  - Metformin (ER 500mg once daily at bedtime)
    - Off-label,
    - Stimulates anit-inflammatory cytokines IL-10, TGF-β
    - stimulates neurogenesis
- Pentoxyphyline (400mg once daily)
  - Off-label,
  - Inhibits pro-inflammatory cytokines IL-1-β, TNF-α
- Sex Hormones –
  - Off-label to regenerate tissue
  - Testosterone (men ~100mg IM weekly, ~50-100mg topically daily, women 1-5mg topically daily)
  - Estradiol (women 1-2mg orally daily, men will make enough of their own)
- Low dose naltrexone – compounded by a compounding pharmacy
  - Multiple mechanisms of action we are not quite sure of
  - Low dose 0.5-7mg daily hits different receptors that high dose 50-150mg daily

And this…

- Strong prescription medications
  - Opioids
    - Palliative care is exempt from the CDC guideline limitations
    - We do not have better alternatives…yet
    - We have opioid receptors in our brains, and low and behold we have plants that produce chemicals that stimulate said receptors – use them
  - Antispasmodics
    - Carisoprodol
    - Tizanidine
    - Diazepam
      - The ONY drug that has both antispasticity and antispasmodic properties
      - Wdocpharm
      - ith its antianxiety properties you have 2 birds for 1 stone.
    - And many others

And this…

- Anti-Anxiety medications
  - Trazodone
  - Buspirone
  - Benzodiazepines,
    - yes, there is a higher risk combining opioids and benzodiazepine.
    - But for some patients it is the only combination that works
    - Be informed, be sage
- Sleep aids
  - Trazodone (again, 2 birds, 1 stone)
  - Zolpidem/Eszopiclone
  - Mirtazapine 7.5mg at bedtime

And this...

- Anti-depressants
  - Tricyclics
    - Amitriptyline, nortriptyline
  - SSRI's
    - Sertraline, fluoxetine, citalopram, paroxetine
    - Not your best choice--SSRI's can make neurogenic pain worse
  - SNRI's
    - Venlafaxine, Duloxetine
    - A better choice—S**N**RI's are shown to help improve Neurogenic pain

And this...

- Anti-inflammatory diet
- Regular exercise
  - As much as you can tolerate
  - With VERY gradual increases in duration
  - Remember the old adage from high school, No Pain-No Gain?
    - Throw that out—it no longer applies
    - Now, pain = damage. Do NOT cause more damage
    - Light stressing will improve range of motion without causing damage

And this…

- Every day
  - Get up and get dressed in real going out in public clothes. Not sweats and a Tee
  - Interact with other people, preferably in person, and about subjects other than your pain.
    - Find a coffee group
    - Find a card group
    - Join a local philanthropic/service club
    - Get a HAM radio license visit with the world.
  - If you can not wok find some place to volunteer
  - Do something that centers on others

And this…

- Develop, renew, expand your relationship with your higher power

- Develop, renew, expand your relationship with YOU
  - With your new "normal"
  - Focus on what you CAN do rather than your limitations. We all have limitation to some degree.

- Develop, renew, expand your relationships with family
  - Keep the relationships balanced
  - Give as much as you ask for, or more
  - Be conscious of not becoming a burden
  - On the other hand, accept help graciously when offered freely.

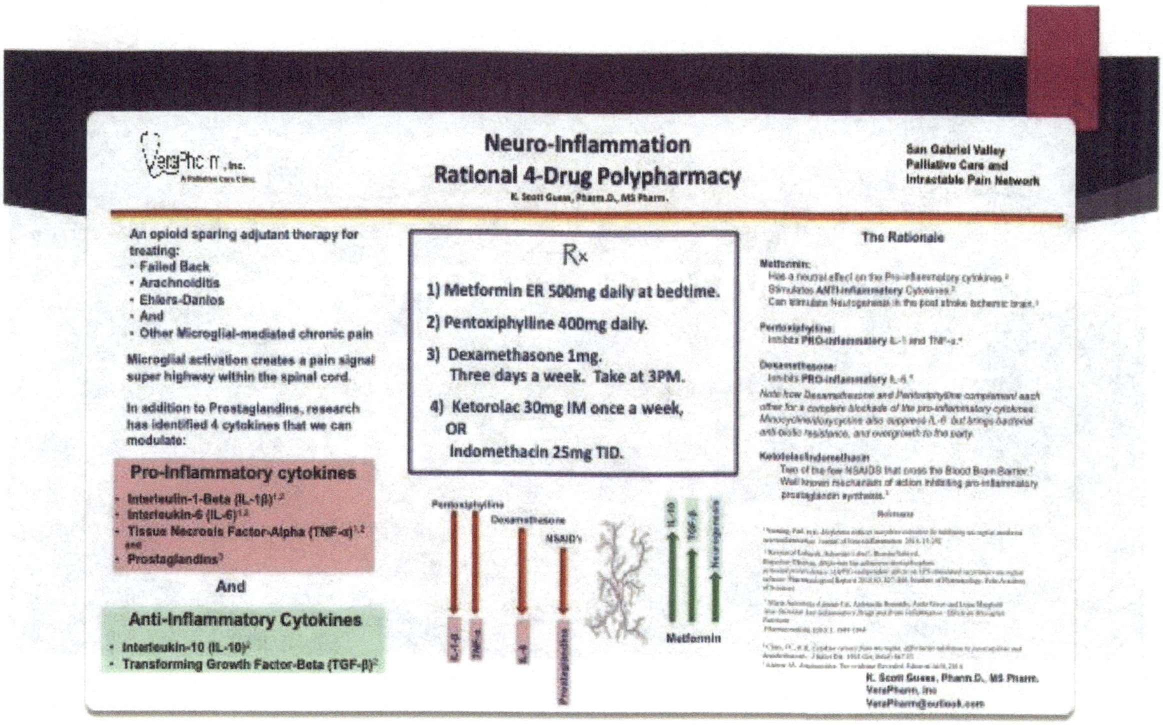
Neuro-Inflammation
Rational 4-Drug Polypharmacy
K. Scott Guess, Pharm.D., MS Pharm.
San Gabriel Valley
Palliative Care and
Intractable Pain Network
An opioid sparing adjutant therapy for treating:
• Failed Back
• Arachnoiditis
• Ehlers-Danlos
• And
• Other Microglial-mediated chronic pain
Microglial activation creates a pain signal super highway within the spinal cord.
In addition to Prostaglandins, research has identified 4 cytokines that we can modulate:
Pro-Inflammatory cytokines
• Interleukin-1-Beta (IL-1β)
• Interleukin-6 (IL-6)
• Tissue Necrosis Factor-Alpha (TNF-α)
• Prostaglandins
And
Anti-Inflammatory Cytokines
• Interleukin-10 (IL-10)
• Transforming Growth Factor-Beta (TGF-β)
Rx
1) Metformin ER 500mg daily at bedtime.
2) Pentoxiphylline 400mg daily.
3) Dexamethasone 1mg. Three days a week. Take at 3PM.
4) Ketorolac 30mg IM once a week, OR Indomethacin 25mg TID.
Pentoxiphylline
Dexamethasone
NSAID's
Metformin
Neurogenesis
Prostaglandins
The Rationale
Metformin:
Stimulates ANTI-inflammatory Cytokines.
Pentoxiphylline:
Dexamethasone:
K. Scott Guess, Pharm.D., MS Pharm.
VeraPharm, Inc

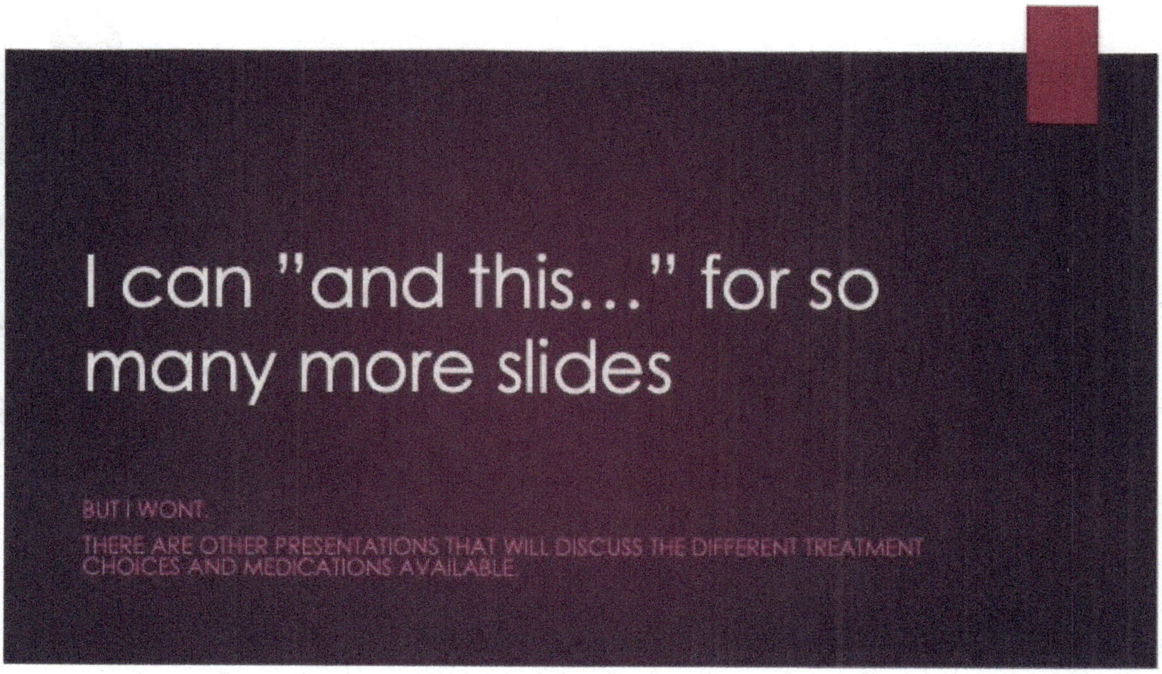
I can "and this..." for so many more slides
BUT I WONT.
THERE ARE OTHER PRESENTATIONS THAT WILL DISCUSS THE DIFFERENT TREATMENT CHOICES AND MEDICATIONS AVAILABLE.

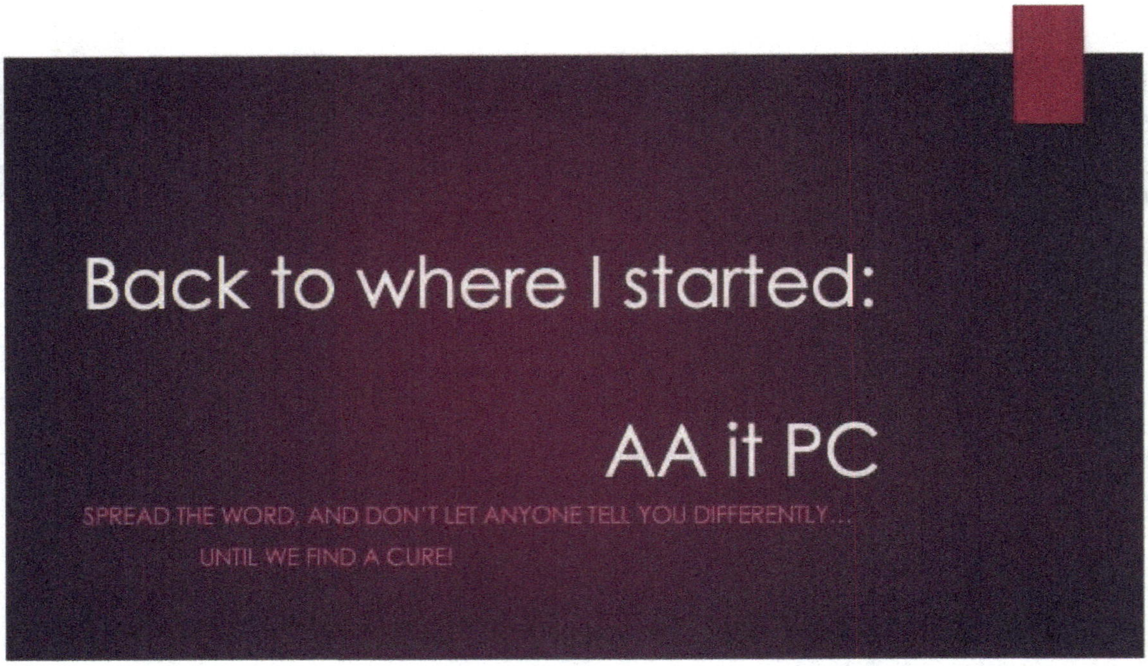
Back to where I started:
AA it PC
SPREAD THE WORD, AND DON'T LET ANYONE TELL YOU DIFFERENTLY…
UNTIL WE FIND A CURE!

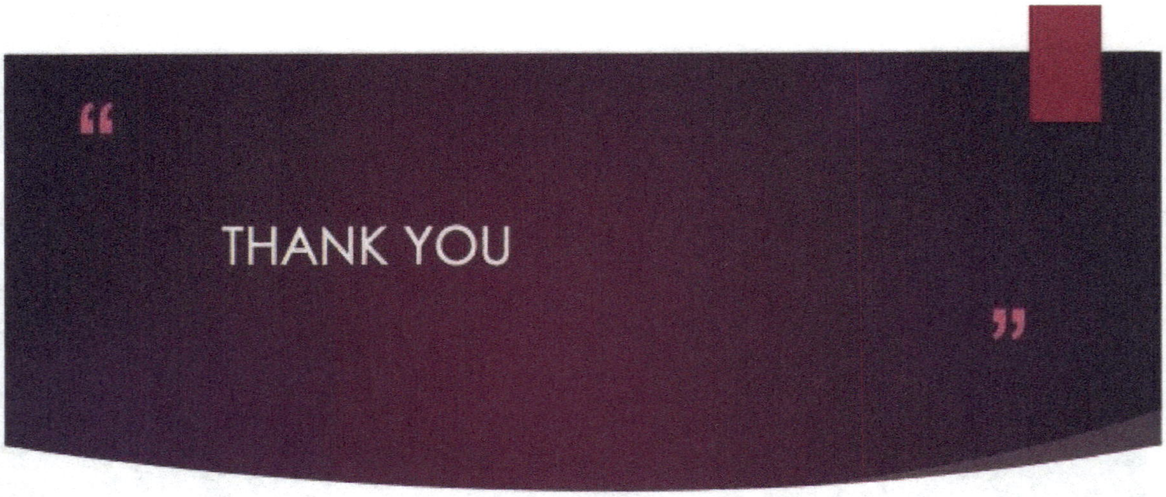
“
THANK YOU
”

ACMCRN- One Team for Arachnoiditis: Advancing Research, Education, and Community: Evelyn Blackburn

This presentation traces the evolving treatment of Arachnoiditis—from the early clinical insights of pioneers like Dr. Antonio Aldrete and Dr. Sarah Smith, to the groundbreaking work of Dr. Forest Tennant, and now toward a new era of collaboration led by ACMCRN.

I'll share how ACMCRN is bridging research, education, and patient advocacy. With tools like the International Patient Registry, a curated physician directory, peer support programs, and community-led awareness campaigns, ACMCRN serves as a hub for uniting patients, researchers, and clinicians to move the field forward—together.

ABOUT ME

Eve Blackburn
Vice President of Patient Engagement,
Arachnoiditis & Chronic Meningitis
Collaborative Research Network
(ACMCRN)

ACMCRN.org

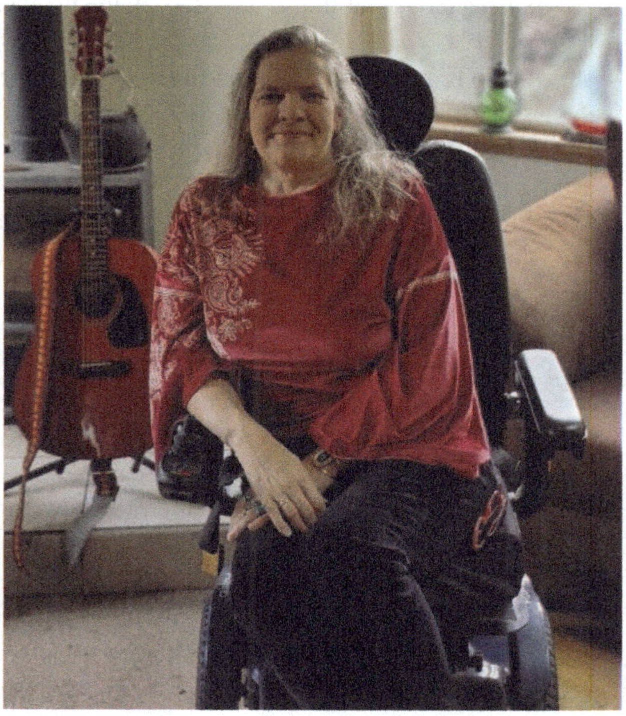

How I Got Arachnoiditis – My Story (Eve Blackburn)

I started in pain management in 1998, after two failed spinal fusion surgeries, and went through a long stretch of invasive procedures. Over the years, I had a pain pump implanted, went through multiple epidural steroid injections (ESIs), and had two different spinal cord stimulators.

In 2009, I was researching my symptoms online when I stumbled on Arachnoiditis. The moment I read the description, I just knew that's what I had. I told my pain specialist, but he dismissed it, saying Arachnoiditis was an "old disease" and there was no way I could have it. Still, he agreed to check.

He performed a CT myelogram, but instead of following standard procedure, he accessed it through the side port of my pain pump—without first clearing the catheter of fentanyl. When he injected the contrast, it pushed that fentanyl straight into my spinal canal and I overdosed.

Amazingly, he continued with the CT while I was overdosing. It took me over a year to recover. He later lied about what happened, claiming it was a cyst at the catheter tip that ruptured and caused the reaction—not the fentanyl.

Fast forward to just last year—during a pump interrogation, they discovered that my catheter is embedded in dense scar tissue, nearly blocking medication flow. While talking to a doctor about what happened in 2009, he confirmed what I'd long suspected—that the "cyst" story made no sense.

I also remembered the pressure shift I experienced during the CT—vomiting, spinning, the whole thing— which was likely caused by the contrast being forced through that scar tissue. That's a separate issue from the overdose, but it all ties in.

I didn't see the CT report until 2016, after I had moved out of state. It simply said: "signs of Arachnoiditis." I'll never forget reading that. The symptoms matched mine exactly. I finally had it confirmed by MRI in 2017, nearly 20 years after the surgeries that likely triggered it.

That's what eventually led me to the Arachnoiditis community on Facebook. Before I joined up with Lori in 2019, I was heavily involved in chronic pain advocacy here in Oregon. I co-founded OPAG (Oregon Pain Action Group) with Wendy Sinclair. We did a lot—testifying, organizing rallies, writing campaigns, media interviews (which I never enjoyed, but did anyway), and pushing back against harmful policies.

Eventually, I hit a wall. The stress, physical strain, and endless hours of work were taking a toll. My body couldn't keep up, so I shifted my focus to advocating for Arachnoiditis—which felt like the right place to put my energy.

Now I live with severe, catastrophic Adhesive Arachnoiditis.

Before all this, in my "old life," I was an office manager, and before that, a certified mechanic. Life has taken some unexpected turns—but I'm still here and still fighting.

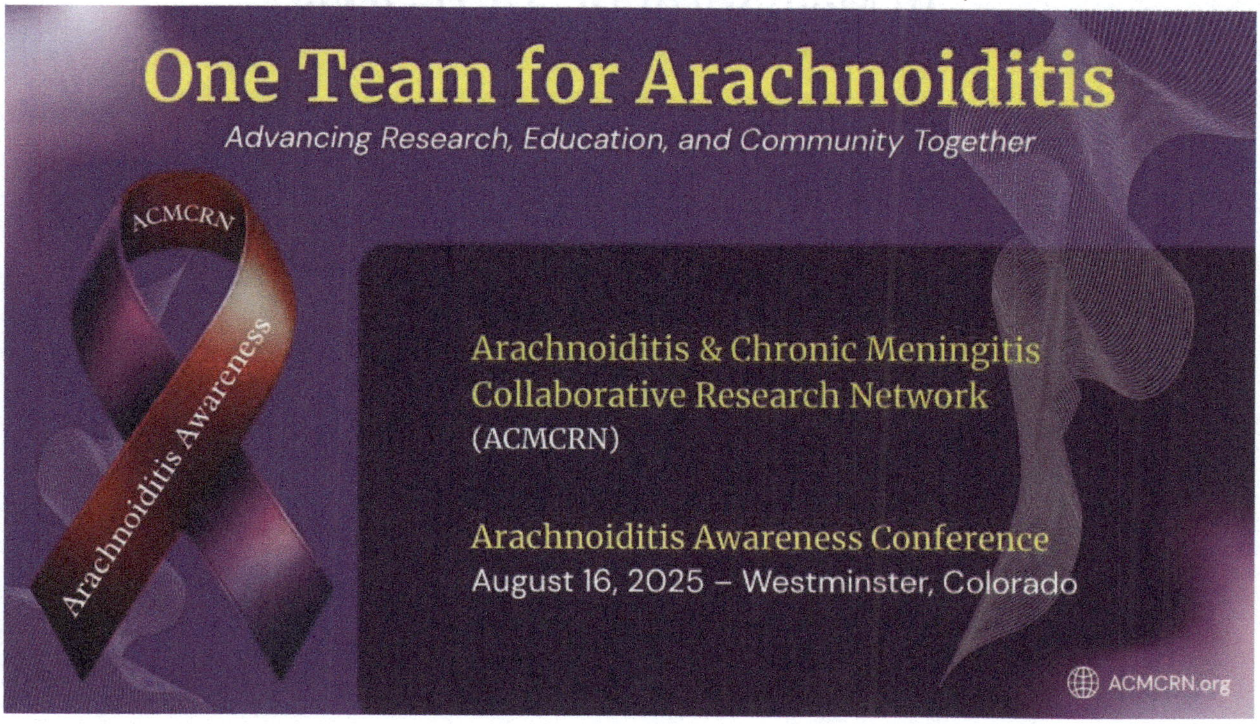

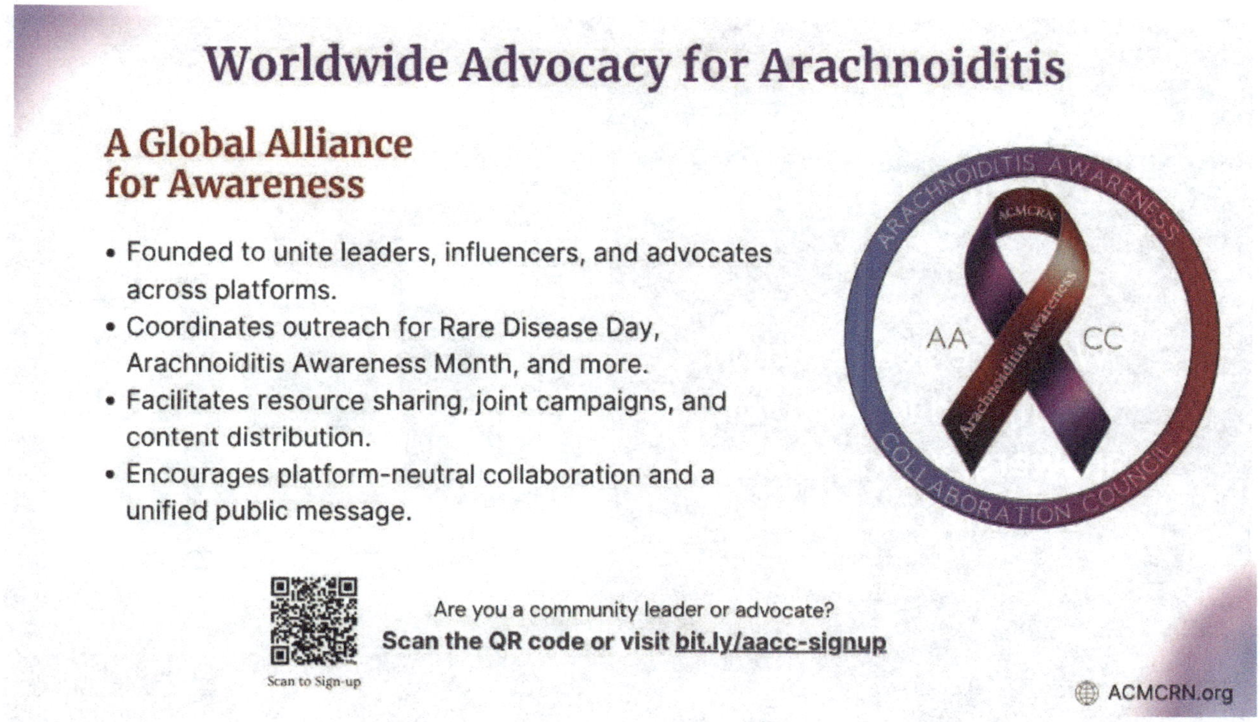

In Memory of Dr. Terri Lewis

Advocate. Educator. Champion.

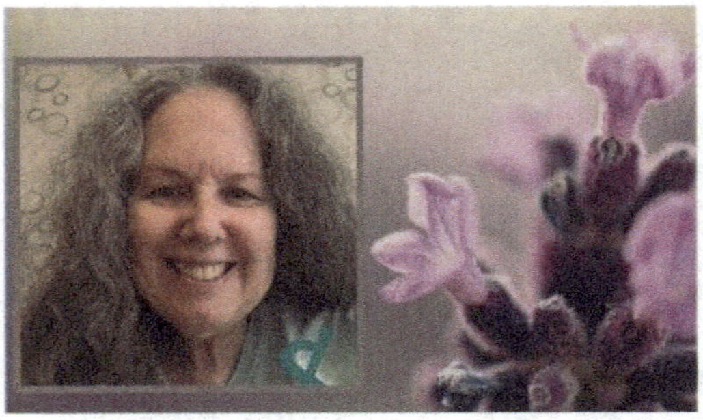

A founding board member of ACMCRN and our first Vice President of Research, Dr. Terri Lewis brought wisdom, courage, and deep compassion to our work.

Her legacy lives on in every patient we support, every research initiative we launch, and every voice we amplify in the fight against Arachnoiditis.

We miss her dearly—but we carry her mission forward.

ACMCRN.org

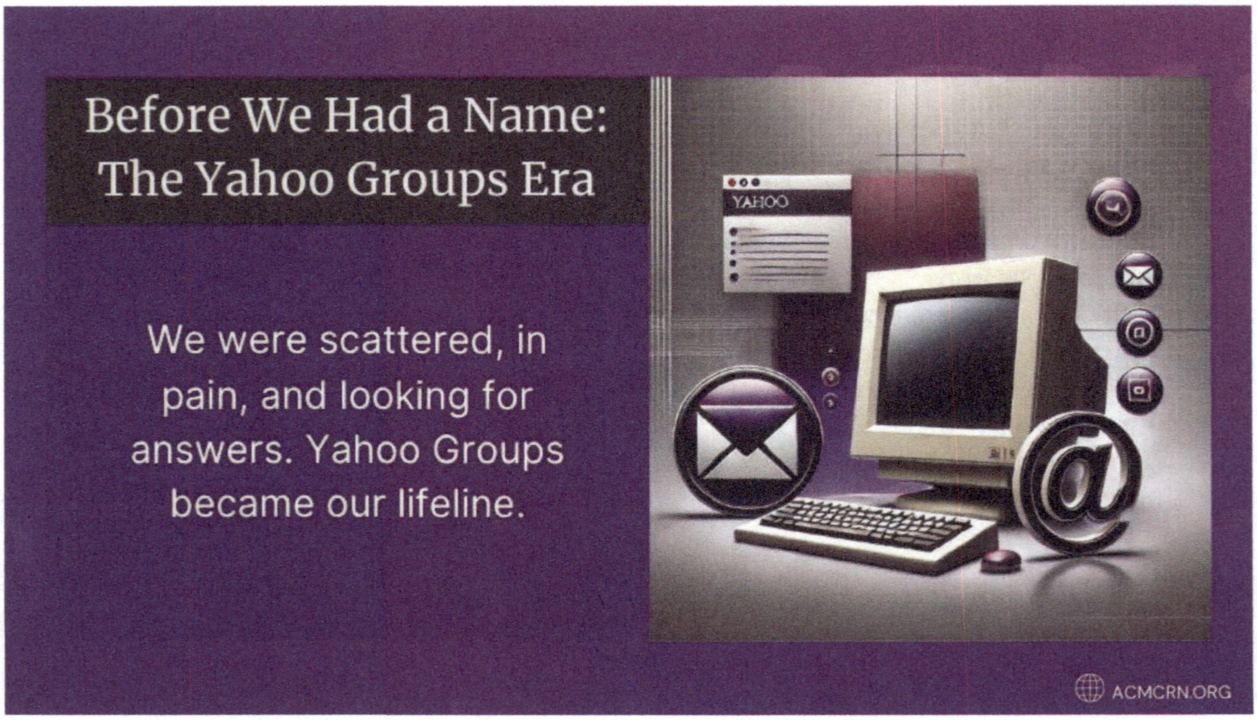

ACMCRN Peer Support Programs

From Isolation to Empowerment

- Weekly Zoom groups for patients, caregivers, and specific needs.
- Special sessions: trauma recovery, life coaching, physiotherapy, and more.
- Safe, inclusive space to share, learn, and grow together.
- Launching the Arachnoiditis Educators program to train peer mentors in rare disease communication.
- Peer Navigators help guide new patients through educational tools, community forums, and treatment options.

Support from someone who understands can change everything.

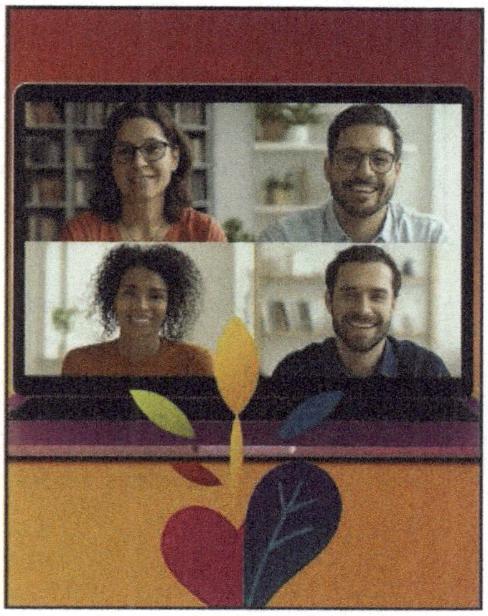

ACMCRN.org

Our Trusted Physician Directory

Crowdsourced. Carefully Managed. Trusted.

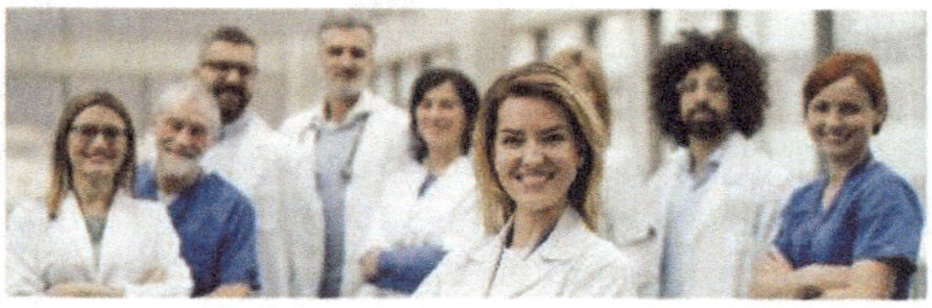

- Our Physician Directory includes over 200 providers: pain specialists, neurologists, physical therapists, alternative therapy providers, and more.
- Curated for over 5 years using community feedback.
- Profiles include notes from patients who have contacted the providers.
- One of the most frequently accessed resources on our website.

Know a doctor who should be included?
Help us grow the directory.
Email: contact@acmcrn.org

Patients helping patients find better care.

ACMCRN.org

Your Gateway to Research, Support, and Community

Visit ACMCRN.org to access research tools, peer support, and advocacy resources.

ACMCRN hosts:

- Research news, events, physician directories, educational videos, PDFs, infographics
- Dr. Tennant's resource archive and curated File Section
- Arachnoiditis Community Forum, live and expanding as a non-social media alternative

Planned upgrades include:

- Tiered membership
- Mailing list scalability (now at 1,500+ members)
- Custom AI-powered chatbot for patient support

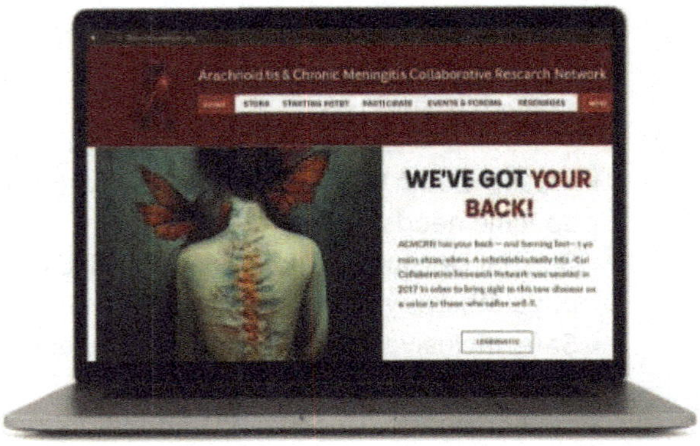

ACMCRN.org

International Arachnoiditis Patient Registry

Real-World Data, Global Impact

- A secure digital research platform owned by ACMCRN and hosted on DigitalCabinet.
- Designed to uncover patterns in neuroinflammation, chronic infections, and patient-reported outcomes.
- Fully compliant with Good Clinical Practice and international ethical standards.
- Patients maintain ownership of their data—consent is required for any use.
- Scheduled to reopen in September 2025 with two new IRB-approved studies.

DigitalCabinet

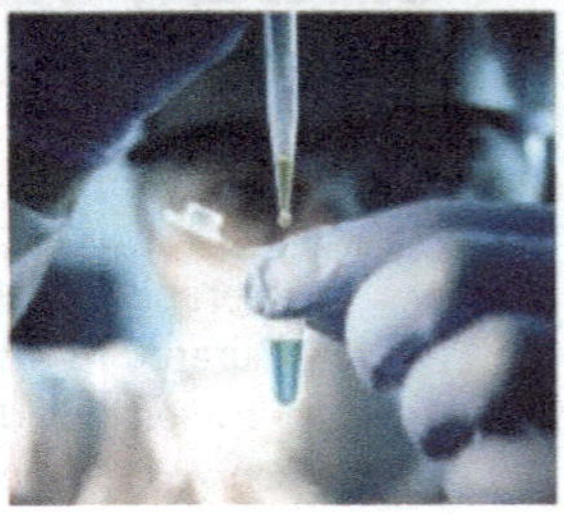

ACMCRN.org

Turning Patient Experience Into Published Science

Global Surveys, Scientific Posters, and a New Research Era

- Vetted patient cohorts available for collaboration
- Survey via StuffThatWorks included 1,250 participants
- Poster presented at 7 international conferences (2023)
- Manuscript nearing submission to an open-access medical journal
- Highlights key findings, research priorities, and future directions
- Aims to increase awareness and attract medical collaborators

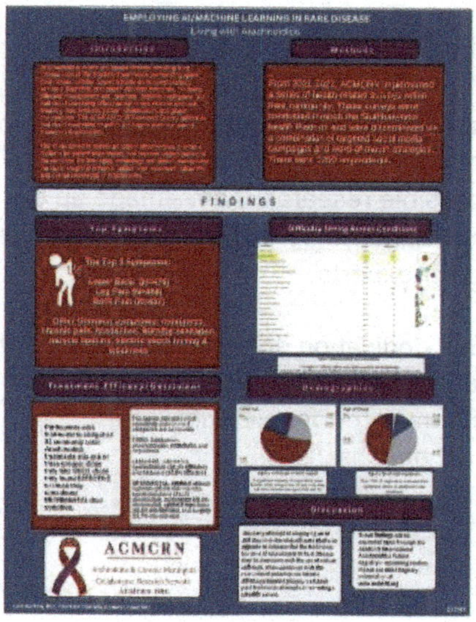

ACMCRN.org

Fueling Progress Together

Every dollar helps sustain our global patient registry, peer support programs, and education campaigns.

Your support covers secure data systems, patient events, and accessible resources—not admin overhead.

Recurring gifts build stability so we can keep showing up for those living with Arachnoiditis.

hope

Together, we're not just funding a project—we're funding hope, answers, and connection.

ACMCRN.org

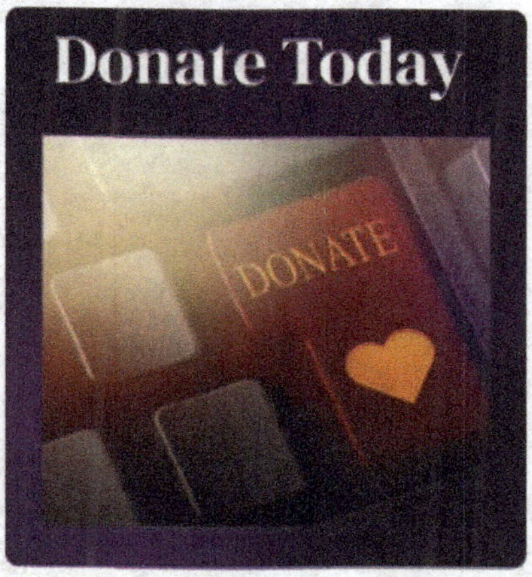

SCAN ME!

Honoring Our Research Team

We proudly acknowledge the leadership of Linda Bavisotto and the contributions of our incredible research team—made up of physicians, an epidemiologist, and subject matter experts.

Their dedication drives every insight, every study, and every step toward better outcomes for people living with Arachnoiditis..

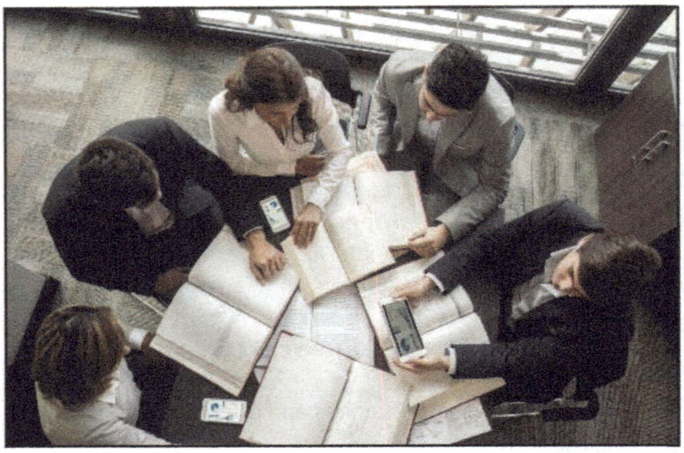

Your work is the backbone of our progress

ACMCRN.org

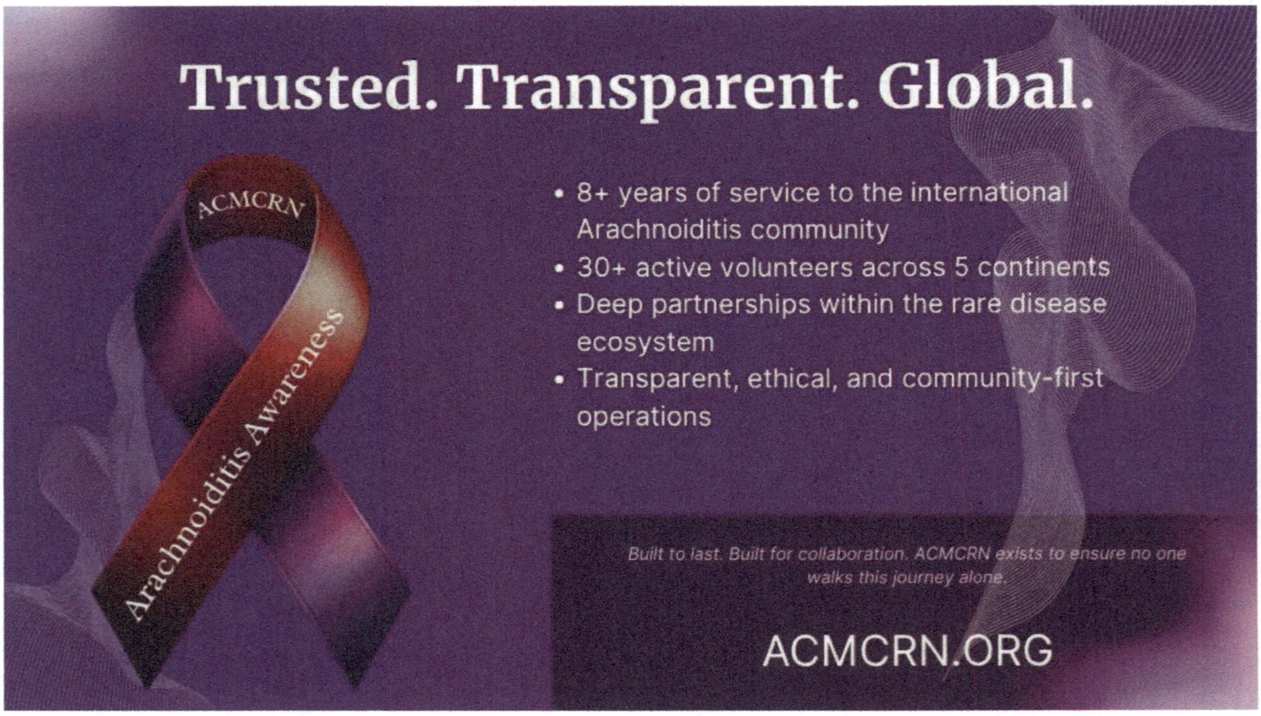

Electro Medical Experience with Frequency Specific Microcurrents (FSM): Amy Marx

I was injured on October 30, 2019, when I picked up a container of laundry detergent in a big box store. There was a defect in the plastic container, and slippery detergent came out of the bottle and onto the floor under my feet. I slammed hard and fast on the concrete floor, on my rear end and ankles. My L4-5 vertebrae shifted as a result, and I now had a spondylolisthesis.

Over time the spondylolisthesis worsened. I developed an odd clenching sensation which worsened and spread throughout my entire lower body. It got so bad that I started to have trouble walking. In the fall of 2022, orthopedists found that the spondylolisthesis was now a level 2, there was no longer a disc, and there was nerve compression. A spinal fusion was recommended. Since nothing, allopathic or alternative had had any effect, I proceeded.

On July 29, 2023, a pre-eminent surgeon at a world-class teaching hospital performed a spinal fusion, discectomy, nerve decompression, and laminectomy. I was given a 90% likelihood of success. Unbeknownst to me, he had seen the Arachnoiditis but had not told me. His thinking was "Well there's no cure for that, but I can do something for this, so I will do a fusion." I was not given the information with which to make an informed decision. Nor was I warned in any way of any risks. It seems he never asked himself if a surgery might make the arachnoiditis worse, which it did, much worse and rapidly.

The surgery left me numb in my private parts, my right buttock cheek, and down the back of my right thigh. I lost all bladder and bowel function. By October 2023 I could barely move my legs. I was housebound and essentially mostly bed bound. I was the worst of the surgeons 1500 outcomes. One time the pulling and clenching in my lower body was so severe that I fell on the floor. To him my surgery was healing nicely.

On October 10, 2023, I had a top to bottom MRI. The report said arachnoiditis. Exhibit 1 is that MRI. I began researching, found Dr Tennant's Foundation, read the books, took the medications, supplements and did everything it advised.

I joined an Arachnoiditis Facebook group and found a post by Paul Manders who had improved in 3 months using Frequency Specific Microcurrent (FSM). I found it locally and began receiving treatments twice a week starting November 7, 2023. The Kaplan Center lent me a machine that I used 24/7. Within a week and a half, I could walk to the end of my driveway. Within three months I could walk three miles and drive again. By April 2024, I was able to return to work as an outdoor craft vendor one day a week. By July 1, 2024, I got off catheters and was back to working two days a week. I was unable to work for an entire year as it's physically demanding.

In May 2024 I went to see Dr Joe Tilchen at Natural Frequency Health in Scottsdale Arizona. Dr Joe uses 12 machines at once and through trial and error determines which frequencies are optimal and programs the unit accordingly. I believe this is what sets Dr Joe apart. To date to my knowledge, he has helped 5 AA patients recover. Programing is $500.

FSM sends micro-currents of electricity at an amperage close to what our nerves utilize at specific frequencies to targeted parts of the body. One channel is directed to the body part, the other at correcting a specific pathology. Essentially it re-aligns the frequency of the mal-performing cells bringing them back into proper functioning. It is very important in a discussion of FSM to understand that, though a science, choosing the correct frequencies is an art and is critical. Because he uses trial and error, testing frequency pairing after pairing, Dr Joe can find the best pairings at that time for each patient and program their machine accordingly. The patient is treated in entirety, not just with FSM. I also utilize his Bio-scan and drops. I have 7 programs; each made of a series of frequency pairings which I go through every day. I wear the machine all day every day. Frequency 13 is for scar tissue dissolution. It is directed at the arachnoid. My MRI of July 29, 2025, shows the nerve clump has somewhat separated and is no longer attached to the wall of the thecal sac. It's been a year and nine months. It's very slow. I do not think it is possible to positively affect AA without using a machine every day at home. The MEND machine ($1500) has more helpful features than the Custom Care machine.

I am not currently taking any medications. I eat a keto diet. Except for weekends when I get a lot of physical exertion at work, I swim laps for at least 30 minutes daily. It's imperative that I stay in motion as much as possible to avoid increased stiffening. The clenching is still there but it has significantly diminished. I get weekly myofascial massage, do Barnes method myofascial release, visceral massage, hydro-colonic therapy, and pelvic floor massage. I got my life back!!!

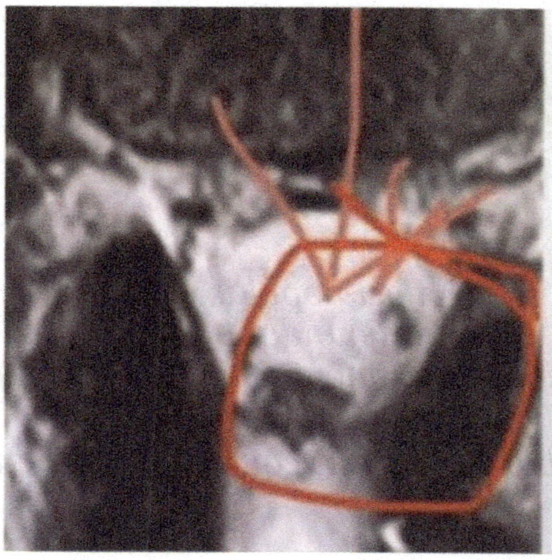

Exhibit 1

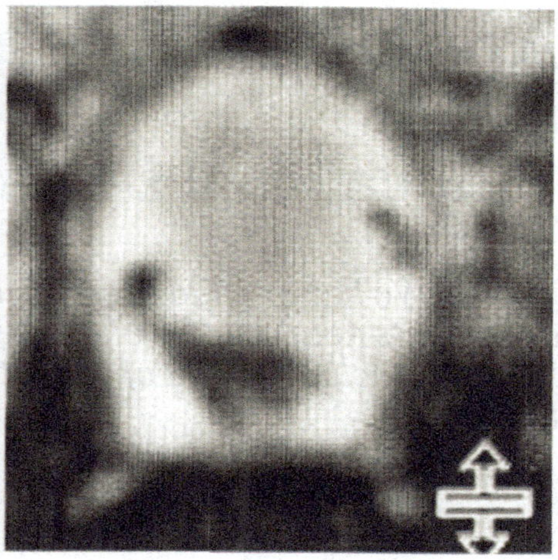

Exhibit 2

Appendix

Educational Documents*

We have included several of the most popular educational documents available through the Tennant Foundation Arachnoiditis Hope. We have included a list of educational documents that have been published to date.

These will be made available by special request by contacting the Foundation.

#2- Daily Protein, Anti-Inflammatory Diet for AA

#15- Exercises for Regeneration and Recovery

#32- Spinal Fluid Flow Exercises

#48- The Relationship Of Epstein-Barr Virus And Adhesive Arachnoiditis - 2025

Tennant Foundation Arachnoiditis Hope
334-338 S. Glendora Ave.
West Covina, CA 91790-3043

Ph: 626-278-4641 Website: www.arachnoiditishope.com Fax: 626-919-7497
Email: tennantfoundation92@gmail.com

Donations can be made via PayPal on our website:

https://arachnoiditishope.com/donations/

Hope

Arachnoiditis Hope

DAILY PROTEIN, ANTI-INFLAMMATORY DIET FOR ADHESIVE ARACHNOIDITIS (AA)

Adhesive arachnoiditis (AA) tends to decrease one's desire for both food and liquids. Rather than prescribe a strict diet, we recommend one that is simple and easy to follow. Protein contains the amino acids that are the building blocks of neurotransmitters and hormones that heal tissues and relieve pain. Protein food(s) must be eaten each day. There are some fruits and vegetables that may suppress inflammation better than others. Some common protein foods and anti-inflammatory fruits and vegetables are listed below.

THE BASIC AA DIET

1. Each day: eat one or more of these protein foods: beef, lamb, pork, poultry (chicken, turkey), seafood (fish, shrimp, crab), cottage cheese, eggs (See Table)
2. Each day: eat some vegetables and/or fruits that may suppress inflammation (See Table)
3. Stop drinks that contain regular sugar (carbohydrates) including fruit juices, soft drinks, coffee, and tea
4. Restrict sugars and starches known as carbohydrates (e.g., breads, pastries, pasta, pizza)
5. Low amounts of alcoholic beverages are permitted

COMMON PROTEIN FOODS	SOME ANTI-INFLAMMATORY VEGETABLES/FRUITS
Seafood: fish, shrimp, crab	Broccoli
Beef	Green beans
Pork	Leafy greens: spinach lettuce, kale
Lamb	Peas
Poultry: chicken, turkey	Corn
Eggs	Blueberries
	Apples
	Oranges
	Pineapple
	Grapes
	Watermelon
	Cantaloupe

At least one serving in each category is required each day.

Note: Persons may wish to supplement protein intake with an amino acid formulation.

This educational information is provided as a public service by "Arachnoiditis Hope" a project of the Tennant Foundation, 336 ½ S. Glendora Ave., West Covina, CA 91790.
Email: tennantfoundation92@gmail.com Fax: 626-919-7497 Website: www.arachnoiditishope.com

#2 Rev 7/25

Educational Document #2

EXERCISES FOR REGENERATION AND RECOVERY

AA Is an inflammatory disease that damages the arachnoid membrane and cauda equina nerve roots. In addition to medications, some exercises will help damaged tissues regenerate and recover. Back muscles and tissues may contract due to pain and spinal fluid seepage.

Our studies and observations of persons with adhesive arachnoiditis (AA) tell us that progressive foot and leg paralysis as well as bladder and bowel dysfunction may develop unless some specific exercises are done each day.

LEG AND ARM EXERCISES (Stand while doing these exercises)

1. Stretch arms straight up and hold for 5-10 seconds. Repeat 3 to 4 times.
2. Raise one knee and leg at a time and hold for 5-10 seconds.
3. Flex your ankle and foot 5-10 times. Can repeat several times a day.
4. Walk with arms swinging only as far as energy will allow. Don't overdo.
5. Stand straight up with legs together. Look slightly upward for 10 seconds (military attention).
6. Stand and rock back and forth on your toes and heels several times a day. (May need to hold on to a chair or cabinet for stability.)

WALKING: Walking is the physiologic cornerstone of AA nerve regeneration. Persons with AA need to take at least two short walks a day (at least 100 feet). Walking upstairs or on a treadmill is excellent.

WEIGHTLIFTING: Lifting a 2-to-5-pound weight is highly recommended twice a day. Simply raising the weight to your body (curls) and raising the weight overhead done on a regular basis will strengthen muscles and other tissues around the lower spine. We believe that light weightlifting done daily will strengthen spinal ligaments and spinal canal cover as well as the arachnoid membrane.

This information is provided as a public service by "Arachnoiditis Hope" a project of the Tennant Foundation, 336 ½ S. Glendora Ave., West Covina, CA 91790.
Email: tennantfoundation92@gmail.com Fax: 626-919-7497 Website: www.arachnoiditishope.com

#15 Rev 7/25

Educational Document #25

SPINAL FLUID FLOW EXERCISES

Spinal fluid in the spinal canal is renewed or "changed over" like oil in a crank case about every 5 to 6 hours. Spinal fluid is a critical body component. It carries nutrients and medicinals to spinal canal tissues including the cauda equina and arachnoid membrane. Equally or more important is that it carries out all toxins, organisms, and metabolic waste that may accumulate in the spinal canal in order to keep the spinal fluid clean, nutritious, and capable of healing.

The micro-masses of AA impede spinal fluid flow. Enhancement or acceleration of spinal fluid flow to keep it flowing at a normal rate helps prevent any infection, contaminant, or metabolic waste from retarding the healing process.

CLINICAL COMPLICATIONS OF FLOW IMPEDANCE BY AA:

We have received numerous reports from persons with AA who have had these manifestations or complications that may be related to spinal fluid flow impedance.

Spinal fluid leaks	Nasal/eye watering	Fainting/falling	Tinnitus
Headaches	Vertigo	Increased cranial pressure	

MAJOR MESSAGE: Exercises to enhance or accelerate spinal fluid flow are simple and some should be done at least once or twice each day by persons with AA to promote healing, and to help prevent deterioration and the complications listed above

SPINAL FLUID FLOW EXERCISES

1. Rocking chair – 5 to 10 minutes
2. Walking or gentle bouncing on a trampoline – 3 to 5 minutes
3. Porch swing, 5 to 10 minutes
4. Deap breathing – hold one minute, repeat 5 to 10 times
5. Arm swings while walking or deep breathing

This information is provided as a public service b "Arachnoiditis Hope" a project of the Tennant Foundation, 336 ½ S. Glendora Ave., West Covina, CA 91790.
Email: tennantfoundation92@gmail.com Fax: 626-919-7497 Website: www.arachnoiditishope.com

#32 Rev 7/25

Educational Document #32

THE RELATIONSHIP OF EPSTEIN-BARR VIRUS AND ADHESIVE ARACHNOIDITIS - 2025

Multiple studies by others as well as our testing and clinical research has compelled us to conclude that the Epstein-Barr virus (EBV) is a causative factor in essentially all cases of adhesive arachnoiditis. Except for autoimmune diseases such as systemic lupus and scleroderma and Lyme disease, we have not been able to identify other causes of chronic inflammation in the arachnoid membrane and cauda equina nerve roots. We now advocate that every person with AA incorporate measures to suppress and eliminate the virus in the treatment program.

The Two Pathologic Mechanisms of EBV: EBV may invade and infiltrate tissues, causing inflammation, tissue destruction, pain, and neurologic impairments. EBV also forms autoimmunity which is the process whereby antibodies or normal cells in tissues are turned into cells that mistakenly attack tissues thinking the tissue is abnormal. The result can be the same as invasion of tissue by the virus: inflammation, tissue destruction, pain, and neurologic impairments.

EBV Reactivation: Anytime a person is in a situation that may diminish or compromise one's immune system, EBV may reactivate from its normal, parasitic existence in lymphocytes. Situations that commonly produce reactivation are severe trauma, including surgery, infections such as pneumonia or meningitis, and severe psychologic stress such as a divorce or bankruptcy. Once reactivated the virus will invade tissue and develop an autoimmune disorder. The reactivation that causes AA may have taken place months or years prior to the development of AA. Initial tissue damage may be in intervertebral discs before the arachnoid membrane. EBV invasion also has a proclivity to invade damaged tissue such as may occur in spinal injuries.

Testing Indicators: EBV produces two main antibodies: viral capsid (VCA) and nuclear antigen (EBNA). Our criteria for clinical action are levels two times normal. VCA represents past reactivation that could cause AA and EBNA likely represents the presence of autoimmunity that is causing the generation of ongoing inflammation. There are two tests for current active infection (early EBNA) and Polymer Chain Reaction/DNA (PCR). If either of these are positive, attempts must be made to suppress the active production of EBV.

Treatment: There are two approaches: suppression and elimination. A number of vitamins, minerals, amino acids, and herbals may suppress future reactivations. Included, but not limited are vitamins C and D, lysine, selenium, zinc, and curcumin. Suppression also seems to occur with monolaurin and thymosin. Elimination is clinically attempted by antiviral agents and ivermectin.

Ivermectin's Growing Popularity: Persons with AA are finding that a short course of ivermectin (2 to 4 weeks) produces pain relief, energy increase, and an enhanced feeling of well-being. Ivermectin apparently acts by eliminating EBV from tissues. At this point, we recommend short trials of ivermectin by persons with AA.

Special Risk Factors: Persons with a genetic connective tissue disease, especially Ehlers-Danlos Syndrome, are prone to EBV reactivation. Persons with a history of infectious mononucleosis may also be prone to reactivation or even carry an autoimmune disorder since the infection.

Educational Document #48

Education Documents Index

These will be made available by special request by contacting the Foundation.

1. How EBV Turns a Spine Injury into Chronic AA
2. Dietary Measures for AA
3. Pathologic Developments and Complications of AA
4. Diagnostic Screening Test for EDS
5. Eight Major Symptoms of AA
6. Screening Test (5 Questions) for EDS
7. Blood Tests for Medical Management of AA
8. Adhesive Arachnoiditis – 2025
9. Palliative Care
10. AA Is a Nerve Entrapment Disease
11. Critical Vitamins and Minerals
12. Peptides In Treatment of AA
13. Non-Adhesive Arachnoiditis
14. Stages and Categorization of AA Severity
15. Exercises For Regeneration and Recovery
16. Maximal Daily Opioid Dosages
17. Non-Opioid Pain Relief
18. The Medrol Test for Inflammation as a Cause of Pain 19. Medical Practitioners Guide for Diagnosis of Lumbar-Sacral AA
20. Empty Sac – What Does It Mean?
21. Neuropathic Pain in AA
22. Multi-Receptor Pain Therapy is Essential
23. Descending Pain
24. Screening Test for EBV Autoimmunity
25. Epstein-Barr Virus Testing for Medical Management of AA
26. Prevention of Epstein-Barr Virus Reactivation
27. Herbal and Natural Medicinals
28. Cervical Arachnoiditis
29. Tarlov Cysts
30. Spinal Fluid Seepage
31. AA and CEID are The Same Disease
32. Spinal Fluid Flow Exercises
33. Spinal Canal Inflammatory Disorder Related to AA
34. Multi-System Disease – Rev 7/25
35. Water Soaking for AA

36. Special Hydromorphone Formulation
37. Peptide Resources
38. Association of EDS and AA
39. How Lumbar Punctures, Epidural Injections, and Surgery Cause AA – 8/25
40. Low Dose, Ketorolac and Methylprednisolone
41. Diagnostic Screen for Hypermobile Spectrum Disorder/Collagen Deficiency Diseases
42. Maximal Medical Treatment for IP
43. Emergency and Flare Treatment
44. Basic Protocol for ARC – Rev 8/25
45. Necessity of 3-Component Protocol for AA
46. Treatment Evaluation Categories
47. Two Phases of Treatment: Stabilization, Curative 8/25
48. The Relationship of Epstein-Barr Virus and Adhesive Arachnoiditis- 2025

Books by Dr. Forest Tennant:

Dr. Tennant's books are available through Amazon/Kindle. They are highly recommended for patients, family, and medical practitioners. Use link provided below for ordering books/Kindle on Amazon.*

1. 2nd Edition "Handbook for New Cases of Adhesive Arachnoiditis" – Steps for Treatment
2. Handbook for Epstein-Barr Virus: Testing and Treatment in Severe, Chronic Pain Conditions
3. The Epstein-Barr Virus: A New Factor in the Care of Chronic Pain
4. The Ehlers-Danlos/Arachnoiditis Connection
5. Handbook for Intractable Pain: Recognition and Treatment
6. The Strange Medical Saga of John Henry (Doc) Holliday
7. Handbook for Newly Diagnosed Cases of AA
8. The Strange Medical Saga of John F. Kennedy
9. Clinical Diagnosis and Treatment of AA
10. Handbook to Recognize AA by MRI
11. Intractable Pain Patients Handbook for Survival
12. The Strange Medical Saga of Elvis Presley
13. The Strange Medical Saga of Howard Hughes
14. Adhesive Arachnoiditis: An Old Disease Re-Emerges in Modern Times
15. Handbook to Live Well with Adhesive Arachnoiditis

*Link for Dr. Forest Tennant's books on Amazon/Kindle:
https://www.amazon.com/stores/Forest-Tennant/author/B091J15RBR?ref=ap_rdr&isDramIntegrated=true&shoppingPortalEnabled=true

Tennant Foundation

Contact Information

The Tennant Foundation Arachnoiditis Hope will gratefully accept donations for the "Adhesive Arachnoiditis Study Project."

Send to this address:

**Tennant Foundation Arachnoiditis Hope 336 1/2 S. Glendora Ave.
West Covina, CA
91790-3043 (501 C-3
#95-43535110)**

To donate using PAYPAL go to Arachnoiditis Hope website:
https://arachnoiditishope.com/donations/

Ph: 626-278-4641
Fax: 626-919-7497
Email: tennantfoundation92@gmail.com

Website: www.arachnoitishope.com

Disclaimer: This publication does not contain medical/health advice. The medical/health information is provided for general informational and educational purposes only and is not a substitute for professional advice. Accordingly, before taking any actions based upon such information, we encourage you to consult with the appropriate professionals. We do not provide any kind of medical/health advice. The use or reliance of any information contained in this publication is solely at your own risk.

Made in the USA
Monee, IL
02 November 2026

67385372R00059